COLLABORATION ACROSS HEALTH RESEARCH AND MEDICAL CARE

To our students

Collaboration across Health Research and Medical Care
Healthy Collaboration

Edited by

BART PENDERS
Maastricht University, the Netherlands

NIKI VERMEULEN
University of Edinburgh, UK

JOHN N. PARKER
Arizona State University, USA

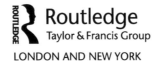

Routledge
Taylor & Francis Group

LONDON AND NEW YORK

First published 2015 by Ashgate Publishing

Published 2016 by Routledge
2 Park Square, Milton Park, Abingdon, Oxon OX14 4RN
711 Third Avenue, New York, NY 10017, USA

Routledge is an imprint of the Taylor & Francis Group, an informa business

British Library Cataloguing in Publication Data
A catalogue record for this book is available from the British Library

The Library of Congress has cataloged the printed edition as follows:
Penders, Bart.
  Collaboration across health research and medical care : healthy collaboration / by Bart Penders, Niki Vermeulen and John N. Parker.
    pages cm
  Includes bibliographical references and index.
  ISBN 978-1-4094-6094-7 (hardback)
1. Medical care–Research. 2. Cooperation. I. Vermeulen, Niki. II. Parker, John N. III. Title.
RA394.P44 2015
362.1072–dc23

2014030615

ISBN 9781409460947 (hbk)

Contents

List of Figures and Tables

Figures

Tables

List of Contributors

Mathieu Albert is Associate Professor in the Department of Psychiatry and Fellowship Programme Director of the Wilson Centre for Research in Education in the Faculty of Medicine at the University of Toronto, Canada. His current work primarily focuses on multidisciplinary relationship between academics and struggle for scientific authority in health research. He has published in a wide range of disciplinary and interdisciplinary journals in social science and in medicine, including articles on symbolic boundaries between scientific groups, science policy-making processes, academic assessment criteria, and funding agencies. He received the Sociology of Knowledge and Technology Section Best Paper Award in 2011 for his paper entitled *Boundary-Work in the Health Research Field: Biomedical and Clinician Scientists' Perceptions of Social Science Research* (Minerva, 2009).

Frans Feron is Professor of Social Medicine – in particular Child and Adolescent Health – and Head of the Department of Social Medicine at Maastricht University, the Netherlands. He has a background in medicine, is trained as a medical doctor (MD), with an official registration as a medical specialist in Community Health and Social Medicine in the field of Child and Youth Health Care. He has over 30 years of expertise in preventive primary care for children and adolescents at the Youth Health Care Division of the Regional Public Health Service, South Limburg. He holds a PhD in Medicine from Maastricht University, where he completed his dissertation based on studies on neurodevelopmental issues in children. His current research activities focus on health, growth and development of children and adolescents, in particular mental health and behavioural problems respectively, and (neuro)developmental issues in children and adolescents.

Claes-Fredrik Helgesson is Professor of Technology and Social Change at Linköping University, Sweden. His research interest concerns in broad terms the intertwining of economic organising, science and technology. The theoretical inspiration comes primarily from economic sociology and social studies of science and technology (STS). His current project 'Trials of Value', together with Francis Lee, investigates the designing of controlled medical experiments as a site where scientific, medical and economic aspects are deliberated upon when establishing what knowledge is worth pursuing. Helgesson is co-founder and co-editor of *Valuation Studies*, a new open access journal, which published its first issue in spring 2013. He is co-editor with Isabelle Dussauge and Francis Lee of *Valuographies: Studies of Value Practices in the Life Sciences and Medicine* (forthcoming, Oxford University Press, 2014).

Brian D. Hodges's research focuses on various aspects of health professional education and practice: competence, assessment, professionalism, and globalisation. He is currently undertaking a three-year SSHRC-funded project together with colleagues at McGill University to study excellence, diversity, and equity in Canadian medical schools' admissions processes. He is an active teacher and speaker, both in Toronto and internationally, on qualitative methods, discourse analysis, and various dimensions of competence. He leads the AMS Phoenix Project, a five-year initiative to rebalance compassion with the technical aspects of healthcare.

Klasien Horstman was trained as a philosophical and historical sociologist at the University of Groningen, the Netherlands. Her master's thesis dealt with the socio-historical context of the rise of the pragmatist philosophy of language. Her PhD, at Maastricht University, addressed the growing role of predictive and preventive medical expertise and technology in life insurance. Her work since has focused on preventive health technologies. To understand the sciences and cultures of prevention, she works at the interface of philosophy, sociology, and science and technology studies. Between 2001 and 2009 she was an associate professor in Maastricht as well as Socrates Professor in Philosophy and Ethics of Bioengineering at Eindhoven University of Technology. During these years she worked on a number of projects focusing on the ethical and societal consequences of genetic and biomedical technologies. Since 2009 she has been Professor of Philosophy of Public Health at Maastricht University.

Linus Johansson Krafve is a PhD candidate at the Department of Thematic Studies – Technology and Social Change, Linköping University, Sweden. He is interested in economic valuation practices in the public sector and its effects on the relations in and between politics, administration, and citizens. His dissertation is about the design of a primary care market in a Swedish county council.

Suzanne Laberge is Professor in the Department of Kinesiology at the University of Montreal, where she teaches sociology of sport and physical activity. She first attained a PhD in anthropology and further decided to undertake an MSc in kinesiology to contribute to the sociological understanding of the health, physical activity, and sport domain. Her research in anthropology and in kinesiology draws mainly on Pierre Bourdieu's social theory. She has published various papers on the study of 'healthy lifestyle' and sport through the lens of Bourdieu's concepts of habitus and field. Her experiences in a multidisciplinary department (kinesiology) lead her to participate with Mathieu Albert on a research project on interdisciplinary collaboration in the health research domain in Canada. More specifically, she investigates how the different health scientists' position regarding the current promotion of interdisciplinary research relates to stakes at the epistemological, disciplinary, and field dynamic levels.

Inge Lecluijze holds a Master's degree in Health Sciences Research from Maastricht University, the Netherlands. She is currently conducting research as a PhD candidate at Maastricht University, studying the implementation process of a novel ICT infrastructure in Dutch child welfare. Drawing on insights from Science and Technology Studies, she investigates how the implementation of a new ICT tool relates to the construction of 'children at risk' and how such an innovation trajectory affects the relationships and trust between State, professionals, parents and children, and the quality of care for youth. Inge is mainly doing research at the interface of technology, politics, science, and professional practices. She is especially interested in the way ICT infrastructures are constructed, processes of implementation, and how new technologies affect professional practices, especially in the fields of child welfare and public health.

Benjamin Lewin is Associate Professor of Sociology at the University of Puget Sound. He is a medical sociologist and his current research explores the intersection of pharmaceutical direct-to-consumer advertising and physician–patient interactions. Advertising of prescription pharmaceuticals is ubiquitous in the United States. Professor Lewin explores the ways in which these ads are reframing the traditional physician–patient relationship into a consumer/exchange relationship that threatens physician authority and autonomy.

Pauline Mattsson is a biotechnology engineer and economist by training. She is a researcher at Karolinska Institutet, Sweden and in 2014 a visiting researcher at Sloan School of Management, MIT. Since 2012 she has been serving as the Vice-President of Euroscience. Pauline has extensive experience from the policy world and has worked for the European Commission and for an innovation policy consultancy, Technopolis Group. She has been a visiting researcher at the Social Science Research Centre Berlin (WZB). Her research is mainly focused on issues related to knowledge transfer and diffusion, innovation systems, innovation, and science/technology policy, especially in the life science and medical technology sectors.

Jessica Mesman is Associate Professor in the Department of Science and Technology Studies at Maastricht University, the Netherlands. Her research interests include the anthropology of knowledge practices and their spatial and temporal dimensions. Her current research has its focus on the exnovation of unarticulated dimensions of patient safety in intensive care practices while using the method of video-reflexivity.

Koichi Mikami is a research fellow of the Wellcome Trust-funded project 'Making Genomic Medicine' at the Science, Technology and Innovation Studies (STIS) Department of the University of Edinburgh (UK). He obtained his D.Phil from the University of Oxford (UK) and, prior to joining STIS, he held the position of an assistant professor at the Graduate University for Advanced Studies in Japan, where he conducted the study of regenerative medicine research. His research interest lies in the relationship between the trajectories of biomedical research and its socio-material infrastructure.

John N. Parker is a fellow at Barrett, the Honors College at Arizona State University. His research focuses on social dimensions of scientific work, scientific elites, social movements in science, science–policy interactions, and the role of emotions in scientific thinking and small group creativity. He also likes to paddle canoes, camp, and is attempting to learn the ukulele.

Bart Penders holds degrees in Molecular Biology and Science and Technology Studies. He is currently Assistant Professor in Biomedicine and Society, researching and teaching at Maastricht University, the Netherlands. In 2013–2014 he was also Edmond J. Safra Network Fellow at Harvard University. In previous years, he was a visiting scholar at Bielefeld University, Germany, and the University of Canterbury, Christchurch, New Zealand, and a postdoctoral research fellow at the Centre for Society and the Life Sciences, Radboud University, Nijmegen, the Netherlands. His research deals with collaboration in biomedicine and nutrition. He studies how scientists and professionals collaborate to create knowledge, how they render such knowledge credible and how non-scientists are involved in both knowledge production and knowledge credibilisation.

David Schleifer researches and writes about food, healthcare, technology, and education. David has conducted research at organisations including Columbia University Medical Center, the New York City Department of Health, the Hunger Project, the National Gay and Lesbian Task Force Policy Institute and the Oregon Social Learning Center. He holds a Bachelor's degree in Sociology from Wesleyan University and a PhD in Sociology from New York University, where he wrote his dissertation about how and why food corporations invested in replacing trans fats. David was the John C. Haas fellow at the Chemical Heritage Foundation in 2008–2009 and a science policy writing fellow in 2012–2013 at Arizona State University's Consortium for Science, Policy and Outcomes. He is currently Senior Research Associate at Public Agenda in New York, a non-partisan, non-profit research and engagement organisation. The views expressed here are not necessarily those of Public Agenda or its funders.

Niki Vermeulen specialises in science and innovation policy and the organisation of research, with an emphasis on scientific collaboration in the life sciences. She is a lecturer in history/sociology of science in the Science, Technology and Innovation Studies subject group of the University of Edinburgh, and her current research project on the emergence of systems biology is supported by the Wellcome Trust. Niki holds a PhD in Science and Technology Studies from Maastricht University (the Netherlands), was a Marie Curie research fellow at the Science and Technology Studies Unit of the University of York, researcher and lecturer in the Department for Science and Technology Studies, University of Vienna (Austria), and research fellow at the Centre for the History of Science, Technology and Medicine of the University of Manchester.

Andrew Webster is Professor in the Sociology of Science and Technology, with a special interest in biosciences and health technologies and the development of emergent fields in the life sciences more generally. He is Director of the Science and Technology Studies Unit (SATSU) at the University of York, Chair of the Economic and Social Research Council (ESRC) Doctoral Training Centre (DTC) combining York, Leeds and Sheffield, and PI on a new (2014–2017) ESRC research project on innovation dynamics and clinical uptake in regenerative medicine (£1.3m). He is also Chair of the European-funded COST Action on 'Bio-Objects' which explore the scientific, innovative, and regulatory aspects of novel biological 'objects', such as stem cells, transgenics, and synthetic biology. He was Dean of Social Sciences at York between 2009 and 2013, and Head of the Department of Sociology 2005–2009. SATSU was an EU-funded Marie Curie PhD training site between 2001 and 2005, and was also responsible for coordinating the UK Stem Cell Initiative (2005–2009) and the FP7-funded regenerative medicine in Europe (REMEDiE) project (2009–2013).

Acknowledgements

We extend our sincere gratitude to all those who contributed to the formation and completion of this volume. This volume was born out of a triple session on 'Collaboration across Health Research and Care' at the 2011 Society for the Social Studies of Science (4S) Annual Meeting in Cleveland and we thank all those involved in those sessions – as contributors and as discussants. We thank our current and former host institutions who provided us with an academic home when we prepared the book. We also thank the Centre for Society and the Life Sciences in Nijmegen, the Netherlands, for supporting our ongoing project by granting visiting scholarships to John N. Parker and Niki Vermeulen and for supporting the workshop 'Collaborations in the Health Sciences', 6 July 2011. We owe gratitude to the reviewers of all the chapters, for their willingness to critically contribute to their quality, as well as the anonymous reviewers of the volume, who helped us to tighten and improve it. We especially thank our editor, Neil Jordan, and supporting staff at Ashgate, who have guided us for the second time, adding another volume to our explorations of collaboration. Finally, we thank all the researchers, clinicians, physicians, nurses, and other medical and health care staff for their willingness to participate in the collection of studies that lies before you.

PART I
Introduction

Chapter 1

When Scientists, Scholars, Clinicians, Physicians and Patients Meet

Bart Penders, John N. Parker and Niki Vermeulen

In 2011 a patient died as a result of poor collaboration between pulmonary surgeons in the Free University Medical Centre Amsterdam.[1] Such fatalities are not unheard of. The Dutch hospital 'De Sionsberg' was forced during the same year to close its cardiology department following a report by the Dutch Association for Cardiology noting that since 2009 the quality of collaboration between cardiologists, management, other specialists, and hospital staff had been consistently poor. Closure was a preventative decision made by the hospital board to avoid fatalities as a result of improper care.[2] Similarly, the cardiology department of University Hospital St. Radboud was shut down in 2006 because of unexpectedly high mortality rates. Again, the closure was not relatable to any one person's actions. As the attending report notes, 'The heightened mortality and morbidity cannot be attributed to the shortcomings of one individual or one group in the cardio-surgical chain of care'.[3] In the United Kingdom, the Mid Staffs Hospital scandal – possibly associated with deaths of 400–1,200 patients over the course of five years due to a low level of care – was, amongst many other things, attributed to insufficient governance of the diverse professionals that ought to contribute to care.[4] The safety and quality of care is thus closely intertwined with the organisation of care work and the ways in which carers work together.

These examples cover a few hospitals over the period of a few years, but let them stand in for many others. Our purpose is to highlight the expectation that health care professionals are expected to collaborate together as harmoniously and as efficiently as possible by the health inspectors, peers, managers, subordinates, the general public, and representatives of the people. Failure to do so may result in

---

1   See: http://medischcontact.artsennet.nl/actueel/nieuws/nieuwsbericht/106879/igz-vumc-reageerde-slecht-op.-calamiteit.htm.

2   The report is available online, see: http://www.skipr.nl/actueel/id7746-ziekenhuis-dokkum-onder-verscherpt-toezicht-.html and http://www.skipr.nl/actueel/id8242-de-sionsberg-sluit-cardiologie-vier-weken.html.

3   See: http://www.onderzoeksraad.nl/uploads/items-docs/364/rapport_hartchirurgie_sint_radboud.pdf.

4   See: http://www.theguardian.com/society/2013/feb/06/mid-staffs-hospital-scandal-guide?guni=Article:in%20body%20link.

sanctions for specific individuals, or at a collective level into fines or even closures for hospitals, departments, and care organisations, to say nothing of insalubrious consequences for public health and for public trust in the healthcare system.[5] Unsurprisingly, calls for expanding and enhancing collaboration in health care are regularly expressed, and increasingly promote the use of information technologies to realise 'better collaboration'.[6]

Collaboration is part of the archetypical image of the medical professional, health care, and social worker and is an elemental aspect of contemporary medical practice. Physicians, specialists, nurses and supporting staff are expected to operate as a well-oiled team. Even the family doctor, seemingly alone at her desk, must communicate, coordinate, and cooperate with apothecaries, specialists, and lab workers to provide even the simplest care. And while the health researcher crunching data behind her computer, performing experiments in her lab and reading up on the newest biomedical research on her iPad might be less associated with collaboration, they work within the same complex organisational ecology of health research and health care, although their work, tasks, collaborative profile, forms of social and cultural capital, and expert roles vary significantly from those of other health professionals. This volume works to better illuminate, characterise and problematise this complex ecology blending in various ways and degrees basic science, medical practice, and entrepreneurial activities by exploring different forms of collaboration across a wide variety of subjects, organisations, and national contexts.

This book follows a continuous line of inquiry beginning with our earlier collection *Collaboration in the New Life Sciences* (Parker et al., 2010), which documented the trend towards and reasons for increasingly large, diverse, and complicated forms of collaboration arising in the life sciences. Expanding these considerations into collective work in health sciences and health care, characterised by its own distinctive dynamics, institutional landscapes, and specific political motivations and implications, is a natural next step in the general quest for understanding how, why, and with what consequences knowledge workers conjointly operate in producing, translating, and employing new forms of information and understanding.[7] In collecting studies of collaboration, the volume's chapters tie into existing debates in literature on health sciences, translational research and care, while focussing explicitly on more general

---

5   This occurred at the Ruwaard van Putten Hospital in Spijkenisse. The hospital was passed over by prospective patients because of problems, initially at the cardiology department. It was the first hospital in the Netherlands to go bankrupt, in 2013.

6   See, for instance: http://www.theguardian.com/society/2007/jun/13/publicservices. comment and http://www.rvo.nl/sites/default/files/bijlagen/Minister%20Schippers%20 zoekt%20innovaties%20die%20de%20zorg%20beter%20en%20goedkoper%20maken.pdf.

7   This line of research that we have set-up over the last decade has resulted in separate and shared papers and books, including Parker (2006), Vermeulen (2009), Penders (2010), Parker et al. (2010) and Vermeulen et al. (2013).

processes, structures and patterns of collaboration and collaborative work. As such, we present collaboration as a *modus operandi* for care and research work, or a specific 'way of knowing' which differs from previous and parallel ways.

Collaboration in Health

Historians have described the emergence of large biomedical complexes (Capshew and Rader, 1992; Creager, 1998; Neushul, 1993; Rasmussen, 2002; Seidel, 1992), which represent some of the first forms of complex, large-scale collaboration in health science and care. Collaborations between academic science and the biomedical industry can be traced back to the 1920s and 1930s when American pharmaceutical firms began investigating in research as a competitive strategy aiming to use science to inform therapeutic practice. These firms opened in-house laboratories and turned to university scientists as source of expertise: 'In a typical collaboration, a firm would fund an academic researcher and stipulate that new processes and inventions be patented and assigned, or licensed on favourable terms, to the firm. Royalties to the university hosting the research would be part of the arrangement' (Rasmussen, 2002: 120). In the context of World War II, alongside large-scale physics projects that produced the atom bomb, biomedical projects focussed on the development of penicillin and blood products. After the war the United States government became a leading patron of the expanding life sciences – funded by the National Science Foundation and the National Institutes of Health. Similar developments took place in other countries.

Turning our eye to the present, and painting with a broad brush, the study of collaboration in the health sector can for analytic purposes be separated, into three sets of studies. The first set, in line with studies of collaboration in other scientific fields, illuminates why, how, and in what ways health researchers join forces with each other. Building on De Solla Price's (1965) seminal work on 'big science' and the growth of scientific inquiry, it assesses and measures collaboration through, for instance, quantitative analyses of the number of authors on a publication (Mattson et al., 2008). Such studies describe collaborative patterns in health and medical research, both internationally and regionally (e.g. Chinchilla-Rodríguez et al., 2012), often in connection to specific pathologies, such as stroke (e.g. Dirnagl et al., 2013). Simultaneously, in-depth qualitative empirical analyses of concrete cases explore the dynamics of health research collaboration, including its motivations, dynamics and consequences. Studies within this area also focus on laboratories, clinics, or larger, less tangible international collectives such as the Cochrane Collaboration (McKenzie et al., 2013) or clinical trials (Gennari et al., 2004; Petryna, 2009).

The second set of studies analyses collaboration between health care professionals, with clinics and hospitals as the main site for collaborative work. These studies research both policy and practice, and address themes such as the division of labour and the relative autonomy of diverse (semi-) professionals (e.g. Loxley, 1997; Hudson, 2002), leadership styles, language barriers, organisational boundaries, and the role of protocols and guidelines (e.g. Marshall et al., 1979; Ovretveit, 1990; McGrath, 1991; Leathard, 2003; Paradis et al., 2014). Medical sociology is a prominent source of this type of study (see e.g. Bird et al., 2010, esp. part iii), as are growing numbers of STS researchers studying medical practice and care (Strating et al., 2011; Van de Bovenkamp and Zuiderent-Jerak, 2013). Above all else, these studies highlight the social, political, and moral diversity within health care and their demonstrable effects on the work and infrastructures that shape it and the amount, relevance, and quality of care provided.

Finally, boundaries between research and care are fuzzy, as are boundaries between the institutions responsible for knowledge making and care-giving. A third set of studies spans the boundary *between* lab and clinic, that is, between research and care. Scholarship in this area deals with the interaction of professionals, disciplines, and sectors, and the translation of biomedical knowledge into a context of diagnosis, treatment or care. The concept of translational research – describing the movement of knowledge, data, and resources – can be traced back to the early 1990s, though it took until 2007 for the National Institutes of Health to propose a definition (Rubio et al., 2010). Still, Woolf (2008) commented immediately afterwards that 'translational research means different things to different people' (p. 211). He posited two 'translational researches', one dealing with 'the transfer of new understandings of disease mechanisms gained in the laboratory into the development of new methods for diagnosis, therapy, and prevention and their first testing in humans' and the other with 'the translation of results from clinical studies into everyday clinical practice and health decision making' (ibid.). Consequently, both translational 'researches' require different tools, skills, and resources and happen in different places.

This volume brings together studies of collaborative practice spanning these three sets of literature by investigating collaborations in and across research and care while paying special attention to intersections between these different bodies of literature since collaborations often cannot be confined to one domain. More specifically, within the health sector a rapidly changing landscape presents professionals operating within it with complexities and uncertainties requiring the combination of multiple social roles and collaborations with diverse sets of actors. Consider, for instance, the growing scale of health collaboration, in which large international consortia devoted to medical innovation are established, clinical trials are conducted simultaneously in various countries, and treatment guidelines are pushed globally. These processes are associated with increasing pressure to standardise through protocols or guidelines and increasing adoption of evidence-based medicine, again demanding coordination and collaboration (see e.g. Van de Bovenkamp and Zuiderent-Jerak, 2013). Additionally, and against the background of the data deluge, new collaborative practices form around data collection and annotation, enabling the collective use and reuse of data relevant for health research and care practices (e.g. Leonelli, 2013). Such dynamics in the research landscape and the health care system warrant in-depth analysis of how professionals collaborate, as well as how these dynamics transform the ways in which they collaborate.

Taken together, this volume attends to the diversity of actors, relationships, organisations, and institutions involved in the collaborative health care and research. Next to scientists and caregivers, the stakes are also high for actors ranging from patients to the pharmaceutical industry. Public–private collaboration is prominent when it concerns drug development, but features in domains such as public health and prevention as well. Especially there, it is subject to a lot of critique (Marks, 2013; Roerich et al., 2014). Public–private collaboration also features in concrete care practices on the hospital floor through its products – such as medical devices and drugs with their protocols and guidelines. Other potential collaborators include patients and their organisations, participants in clinical trials, volunteers, and administrators (Douglas, 2012). Moreover, social scientists and ethicists are increasingly welcomed on board as collaborators in both research and care practices. As Andrew Webster elaborates in the final chapter of this book, this diversification ties into the question of who counts as a legitimate collaborator – at the individual as well as institutional level – and where responsibility, accountability, and ownership are situated.

Studying collaboration in health care and research allows us to learn about the ways in which knowledge producers cooperate, generate new forms of practice, and constitute new forms of knowledge and infrastructures to support such knowledge. The studies collected in this book extend our knowledge about the social organisation and content of collaboration precisely because these settings are diverse and join basic and applied forms of research. Furthermore, as the opening lines of this chapter indicate, these subjects are high on governmental agendas and have direct impacts on the life quality of individuals and the success and failures of organisations. The health sector confronts practices of collaboration with a unique constellation: a mix of basic and applied inquiry, as well as proximity to and dialogue with its object of study, and the ethical and political issues that are connected to medical research and health care. As such, it distinguishes itself from other types of scientific collaboration and warrants our close attention in this overview of collaboration in health research and care.

The Collection

The chapters featured in this volume range from studies in either research or care setting to hybrids of both. They study diverse technological and social platforms in the health domain meant to stimulate collaboration, or objects inadvertently doing so; objects as diverse as stem cells, IT systems, trans fats and children and babies at risk (Vermeulen et al., 2012). They feature administrators, nurses, social workers, molecular biologists, social scientists, and clinicians and physicians set again the backgrounds of neonatal wards, registry infrastructures, virology departments and government offices. They all share, however, a perspective on collaboration, collaborators, and collaborative work.

The collection is divided into three parts following this introduction and Pauline Mattson's overview chapter that takes us on a journey through the scientometric landscape of the health sciences. She demonstrates on the basis of co-authorship analyses the rise of collaboration across a variety of different boundaries: disciplinary, institutional, and geographical. As such, her chapter marks a clear starting point as it firmly establishes collaboration as a style of work in the health sector.

The first section of this volume, *Collaboration in Health Research*, contains chapters that move beyond a diagnosis of collaboration as present and growing and instead examine what collaboration looks like in practice – to the people, disciplines, groups, and institutions at play. In Chapter 3, Niki Vermeulen explains how virology is organised and the ways in which virologists build consortia and especially *projects* in an effort to shape collaboration and knowledge production. She argues that this projectification allows for alignment in knowledge production and innovation, but it also limits flexibility by subscribing to one mode of ordering more than to another. In Chapter 4, Mathieu Albert, Suzanne Laberge, and Brian Hodges consider how collaboration between biomedical and clinical scientists on the one hand, and social scientists on the other, is influenced by the former group's perception of the latter. They analyse biomedical and clinical scientists' rationales for being receptive to, ambivalent about, or dismissive of social science research. Their findings indicate that receptiveness flows from exposure and experience, but with severe limits, since social scientists are relative newcomers to the health field in which biomedical scientists and clinical scientists are at the dominant end of the power distribution. In Chapter 5, David Schleifer studies collaborative work on healthy nutrition, demonstrating that collaborations are sometimes built to establish credibility – to convince. When initial claims on the detrimental health effects of trans fats emerged from the Netherlands, the United States' food industry readily participated in a research collaboration to disqualify these claims. However, in the process of collaboration they convinced themselves that the claims about the trans fat health risks were valid, ensuring credibility of results to the entire food industry.

The second section of this volume, *Collaborative Health Infrastructures*, features two chapters focusing on structures or platforms created to facilitate or enable collaboration. In Chapter 6, Claes-Fredrik Helgesson and Linus Johansson Krafve describe the collaborations and interactions that shape and are shaped by clinical registries. They evince how registries link care and research practices through data collection in a network that can best be described as an amalgam of more intense and less intense collaborative relationships, while also serving as a resource for competition. The authors show that by maintaining that paradoxical role, registries maintain their value for those working in and with them. In Chapter 7, Inge Lecluijze et al. analyse another collaborative infrastructure, describing how the Child Index – a Dutch digital registry for children at risk – was designed to foster collaboration in child welfare. They show how the digital system was supposed to discipline users into collaborating according to prescribed rules, but that child welfare professionals – the users of the system – found creative ways to avoid such disciplining. While the digital system was insufficient to discipline users, child welfare professionals continued to collaborate, albeit with little or no reference to the Child Index – allowing them to maintain professional discretion and autonomy.

The third section of this volume, *Collaboration in Health Care*, presents studies investigating collaboration in care. In Chapter 8, Koichi Mikami examines collaborative patterns in regenerative medicine. He demonstrates that while collaborations were motivated by many factors, a main goal was the establishment of legitimacy – the power within a community to define the field and to determine its rules. Mikami shows multiple strategies used by multiple clusters of experts in Japanese regenerative medicine to achieve legitimacy. He argues that a strategy of growing relevance is the demonstration of 'clinical relevance' through by patient participation. In Chapter 9, Jessica Mesman employs an autobiographical approach to describe her involvement in the introduction of video reflexivity in a Dutch neonatal intensive care ward. She discusses her collaboration with clinicians on the ward and how the method of video reflexivity functions as an infrastructure for collaboration and acts as a framework for the construction of collaborative knowledge. Mesman maintains that collaboration is not only something to study, but something to in which to participate to open oneself up to its strengths and weaknesses and learn from it. In Chapter 10, Benjamin Lewin focuses on collaboration between physicians and individual patients, marshalling findings and theory from medical sociology to demonstrate that patients are active agents in the production of medical knowledge. Through collaborating with physicians in, for instance, the diagnostic process, they contribute to treatment and care outcomes. Patients have legitimate expertise to offer to the collaboration, which, in the case of diagnosis, is generally offered in the form of a patient narrative.

Andrew Webster, in the conclusion of this collection, ties together the main lessons from the preceding chapters, arguing that collaboration in health research and health care has to be understood in the context of a changing landscape characterised by several clearly discernable trends. These include the ever-expanding scale of collaboration – professional, disciplinary, organisational, and geographical – and its consequences for the structure of research, the role of funding in the initiation and design of collaboration, the uncertainties associated with collaboration when it comes to responsibility for, ownership of, sanctions and rewards in, and finally, the competition between large collaborative practice and the local, non-collaborative practices of research and care. He maintains that collaborations may centre on biomedical platforms, yet require social platforms to prosper, and that some forms of collaboration (for instance between scientists and social scientists) are better left to grow and mature on their own, rather than vigorously pursued.

While the collection provides us with a score of lessons to better understand collaborative inquiry and collaborative care in the health sector, it also presents new questions – most notably on its final pages – about the future of a field in which collaboration has become the dominant paradigm, but which continues to change due to innovation from within, as well as through changes in our increasingly globalised world. Healthy collaboration means understanding these dynamics and the relations between the knowledge maker and the care giver, the individual patient and the population, as well as those involved in regulation and governance, while respecting that health research and care is about real people. As we are convinced that there is a lot to learn from existing collaborations, and how they organise their work and their practices, this volume is our contribution to understanding and reflecting on collaboration in health research and care.

References

Bird, C.E., Conrad, P., Fremont, A.M. and Timmermans, S. 2010. *Handbook of Medical Sociology, Sixth Edition.* Nashville: Vanderbilt University Press.

van de Bovenkamp, H.M. and Zuiderent-Jerak, T. 2013. An empirical study of patient participation in guideline development: Exploring the potential for articulating patient knowledge in evidence-based epistemic settings. *Health Expectations* (ePUB, ahead of print: doi: 10.1111/hex.12067).

Capshew, J.H. and Rader, K.A. 1992. Big science: Price to the present. *Osiris, 2nd Series*, 7, 2–25.

Chinchilla-Rodríguez, Z., Benavent-Pérez, M., de Moya-Anegón, F. and Miguel, S. 2012. International collaboration in medical research in Latin America and the Caribbean (2003–2007). *Journal of the American Society for Information Science and Technology*, 63(11), 2223–38.

Creager, A.N.H. 1998. Biotechnology and blood: Edwin Cohn's plasma fractionation project, 1940–1953. In: Thackray, A. (ed.) *Private Science: Biotechnology and the Rise of the Molecular Sciences*. Philadelphia: University of Pennsylvania Press, 39–62.

De Solla Price, D.J. 1965. *Little Science, Big Science*. New York: Columbia University Press.

Dirnagl, U., Hakim, A., Macleod, M., Fisher, M., Howells, D., Alan, S.M., Steinberg, G., Planas, A., Boltze, J., Savitz, S., Iadecola, C. and Meairs, S. 2013. A concerted appeal for international cooperation in preclinical stroke research. *Stroke*, 44, 1754–60.

Douglas, C., 2012. Bio-objectification of clinical research patients: Impacts on the stabilization of new medical technologies. In: Vermeulen, N., Tamminen, S. and Webster, A. (eds) *Bio-objects: Life in the 21st Century*. Farnham: Ashgate, 59–68.

Galison, P. and Hevly, B. (eds) 1992. *Big Science: The Growth of Large-Scale Research*. Stanford: Stanford University Press.

Gennari, J.H., Weng, C., McDonald, D.W., Benedetti, J. and Green, S. 2004. An ethnographic study of collaborative clinical trial protocol writing. *Studies in Health Technologies and Informatics*, 107(2), 1461–5.

Hudson, B. 2002. Interprofessionality in health and social care. *Journal of Interprofessional Care*, 16(1), 7–17.

Leathard, A. (ed.) 2003. *Interprofessional Collaboration: From Policy to Practice in Health and Social Care*. Hove, UK: Routledge.

Leonelli, S. 2013. Global data for local science: Assessing the scale of data infrastructures in biological and biomedical research. *BioSocieties*, 8(4), 449–65.

Loxley, A. 1997. *Collaboration in Health and Welfare: Working with Difference*. London: Jessica Kingsley Publishers.

Marshall, M., Preston, M., Scott, E. and Wincott, P. (eds) 1979. *Teamwork For and Against: An Appraisal of Multidiscipliplinary Practice*. London: British Association of Social Workers.

McKenzie, J.E., Salanti, G., Lewis, S.C. and Altman, D.G. 2013. Meta-analysis and the Cochrane collaboration: 20 years of the Cochrane Statistical Methods Group. *Systematic Reviews*, 2, 80.

Marks, J.H. 2013. What's the big deal?: The ethics of public–private partnerships related to food and health. *Edmond J. Safra Working Paper*, 11, http://papers. ssrn.com/sol3/papers.cfm?abstract_id=2268079.

Mattsson, P., Laget, P., Nilsson, A. and Sundberg, C.J. 2008. Intra-EU vs. extra-EU scientific co-publication patterns in EU. *Scientometrics*, 75(3): 555–74.

McGrath, M. 1991. *Multi-disciplinary Teamwork*. Aldershot: Avebury.

Neushul, P. 1993. Science, Government and the Mass Production of Penicillin. *Journal of the History of Medicine and Allied Sciences*, 48(4), 371–95.

Ovretveit, J. 1990. *Co-operation in Primary Health Care*. Uxbridge: Brunel Institute of Organisation and Social Studies.

Paradis, E., Reeves, S., Leslie, M., Aboumatar, H., Chesluk, B., Clark, P., et al. 2014. Exploring the nature of interprofessional collaboration and family member involvement in an intensive care context. *Journal of Interprofessional Care*, 28(1), 74–5.

Parker, J.N. 2006. *Organisational Collaborations and Scientific Integration: The Case of Ecology and the Social Sciences*. PhD thesis, Arizona State University.

Parker, J.N., Vermeulen, N. and Penders, B. 2010. *Collaboration in the New Life Sciences*. Farnham: Ashgate.

Penders, B. 2010. *The Diversification of Health. Politics of Large-scale Cooperation in Nutrition Science*. Bielefeld (D): Transcript Verlag.

Petryna, A. 2009. *When Experiments Travel. Clinical Trials and the Global Search for Human Subjects*. Princeton: Princeton University Press.

Rasmussen, N. 2002. Of 'small men', big science and bigger business: The Second World War and biomedical research in the United States. *Minerva*, 40(2), 115–46.

Roehrich, J.K., Lewis, M.A. and George, G. 2014. Are public–private partnerships a healthy option? A systematic literature review. *Social Science and Medicine*, 113: 110–19.

Rubio, D.M., Schoenbaum, E.E., Lee, L.S., Schteingart, D.E., Marantz, P.R., Anderson, K.E., Platt, L.D., Baez, A. and Esposito, K. 2010. Defining translational research: Implications for training. *Academic Medicine*, 85(3), 470–75.

Seidel, R. 1992. The origins of the Lawrence Berkeley Laboratory. In: Galison, P. and Hevly, B. (eds) *Big Science. The Growth of Large-Scale Research*. Stanford: Stanford University Press, 21–45.

Strating, M., Nieboer, A., Zuiderent-Jerak, T. and Bal, R. 2011. Creating effective quality improvement collaboratives: A multiple case study. *BMJ Quality and Safety*, 20(4), 344–50.

Vermeulen, N. and Penders, B. 2010. Collecting collaborations. Understanding life together. In: Parker, J.N., Vermeulen, N. and Penders, B. (eds) *Collaboration in the New Life Sciences*. Farnham, UK: Ashgate, 3–13.

Vermeulen, N. 2009. *Supersizing Science. On Building Large-scale Research Projects in Biology*. Maastricht, NL: University Press Maastricht.

Vermeulen, N., Parker, J.N. and Penders, B. 2013. Understanding life together: A brief history of collaboration in biology. *Endeavour*, 37(3), 162–71.

Woolf, S.H. 2008. The meaning of translational research and why it matters. *JAMA*, 299, 211–13.

Chapter 2

The Evolution of Collaborations in Health Sciences Measured by Co-authorship

Pauline Mattsson

Introduction

This chapter aims to contribute to the understanding of how research collaborations in health sciences have evolved over the last three decades using bibliometrics as the method for data collection. Bibliometrics consist of a number of methods that can be defined as 'the application of mathematical and statistical methods to books and other media of communication' (Pritchard, 1969). In the late sixties the interest in bibliometrics took a sharp rise. One decade later, when data collection was often still a matter of manual work, different interdisciplinary approaches and models from mathematics and physics, together with sociological and psychological methods, started influencing the emerging discipline. Since the beginning of the eighties, bibliometrics has evolved into its own distinct scientific discipline with a specific research profile, several subfields, and a specific journal: *Scientometrics*. The main reason for this development was the growing availability of large searchable bibliographic databases in parallel with technological developments in high speed computing and data processing (Glänzel, 2001).

The number of scientific publications in all fields has been increasing steadily over the last decades. One of the first studies confirming this trend was conducted by Smith (1958). He observed a growing number of co-authored publications and started to use multiple author papers as an index for collaboration. Since then, co-authorship has become a frequently used indicator for collaboration. Over the last two decades the growth of collaborating papers has been exponential observed by a number of different studies (Adams et al., 2005; NSF, 2008; Glänzel, 2001). In the latest NSF Science and Engineering Indicators report from 2012 it can be read that two-thirds of all articles published in 2012 were co-authored. The number of papers written by authors from different institutions and countries has continued to increase, indicating an increasing knowledge creation, transfer, and sharing among institutions and across national boundaries.

While it is not the aim of this chapter to discuss why researchers seek to collaborate, I will briefly explore different factors that have been identified as important for explaining the increasing rate of collaboration. In a regression analysis carried out by Adams et al. (2005) the increase of co-publications is explained by the rise of public R&D investment, private control of universities, and increased mobility of PhDs. On a similar note Rigby and Edler (2005) argue that the growth of collaborative research owes much to the provision of funding from governments' intent to encourage interdisciplinarity and interactions between different sectors. Bozeman and Boardman (2003) go as far as talking about a new 'era of inter-institutional research collaboration' referring to US science and technology policy moving from decentralised support of small investigator initiated research projects to large scale and oftentimes centralised, block grant-based, multidisciplinary research. In tandem, the scale, scope and diversity of funding programmes has increased and transnational, national and regional initiatives all play important roles. It is also important to mention that the growing involvement of emerging countries on the global scientific stage has contributed to the increase. This is obvious when studying the number of articles published in international peer reviewed journals by authors from Brazil, South Africa and especially China (Mattsson, 2012). Other factors that can help explain the increasing collaboration rate are the growing use of expensive and large-scale instruments. When a research group does not have the required budget needed to purchase instruments it has to find someone with whom to share the costs (Vermeulen et al., 2013). The interdisciplinarity of a field is also a factor which could affect a research group's tendency to collaborate. If the required knowledge cannot be found within the own research group, it has to be attained through external collaboration.

In this chapter, I use bibliometrics to explore three different dimensions of collaboration within the field of health sciences. This includes, first, the study of the structural properties of the co-publication networks including the number of authors and addresses and type of organisation. Second, I study the interdisciplinarity of health sciences through references. Third, I investigate the geography of collaboration through the involvement of researchers from different countries. The chapter starts with an overview of earlier studies investigating similar topics and subsequently presents an overview of bibliometrics as a method to study collaboration and what are the pros and cons and limitations. Next, I present and discuss the results covering the three different dimensions of health science publications. The last section of the chapter summarises and discusses the main results.

Earlier Literature on Co-publications in Health Sciences

In this section I will briefly present earlier literature that reports the three different dimensions of collaboration using bibliometrics as a method. Existing studies have focused on different scientific fields and also included different sub-fields depending on how different scientific journals have been classified. Therefore it is difficult to make direct comparisons between earlier studies and the results presented in this chapter. Earlier studies that have focused on health sciences are limited and hopefully this chapter will in some way contribute to an increasing understanding about the evolution of co-publications within the field.

Structural Dimension

It is not only the number of publications that has increased but also the number of authors involved in each publication. Adams et al. (2005) measured the average author network of publications and found that all scientific fields have increased from an average of 2.5 authors per paper in 1981 (mathematics being the smallest with 1.5 and medicine the largest with 3.3) to an average of 3.9 in 1999 (mathematics being the smallest with 1.9 and physics the biggest with 7.3). The same authors also showed that physics is the field that has grown fastest in terms of number of authors per publication over the years 1981 to 1999. In a report from the National Science Foundation the number of authors in different fields with at least one author from the US over a 20-year period was analysed (National Science Foundation, 2012). It showed that the average number of author names per paper taking all Science and Engineering fields into account grew from 3.2 to 5.6. Focusing on publications within medical science, according to the classification in the Science Citation Index by Thomson Reuters, the number of authors per paper has grown by 62 per cent from 1990 to 2010. It is the field after physics and astronomy that has the highest number of authors involved in a paper. The average number of authors per paper more than quadrupled in astronomy (3.1 to 13.8) while doubled in physics (4.5 to 10.1). Growth in the average number of co-authors was slowest in the social sciences (from 1.6 authors per paper in 1990 to 2.1 in 2010) and in mathematics (from 1.7 to 2.2). In short, papers authored by a single US academic scientist or engineer are becoming an increasingly small minority of the published literature.

Katz and Martin (1997) investigated the number of departments mentioned in the address line of a publication. They found that 40–50 per cent of all publications related to clinical medicine had more departments listed in the address field than the number of authors included. Similar patterns can be seen in other fields but to a lesser degree, biomedical research and physics (10–15 per cent), biology, earth, and space science (5–10 per cent), and chemistry, engineering, and mathematics (<5 per cent). These results suggest that many researchers in clinical medicine tend to hold joint positions with several departments or institutions. For example clinicians carrying out both clinical work at hospitals and research at universities.

The Interdisciplinary Dimension

Differences between basic and applied research have already been discussed in several studies (Frame and Carpenter, 1979; Luukkonen et al., 1992). The conclusion has been that researchers carrying out applied sciences are often more experimentally oriented rather than based only on theories and therefore the need to collaborate is also stronger (Price, 1963; Hagstrom, 1965; Gordon, 1980). The growing use of expensive and large-scale instruments can also help explain the increased collaboration rate. The importance of access to infrastructure to carry out a certain type of research has been growing over the decades due to technological development. When a research group does not have the required budget needed to purchase instruments it has to find someone to share the costs with. These types of collaboration are specifically common in fields such as physics and astronomy where only a few instruments exist around the world, for example the Large Hadron Collider at CERN in Switzerland (a large particle accelerator), or the Pierre Auger Observatory, an international cosmic ray observatory located in Argentina, or large high-Tesla MRI scanners in the medical field.

The interdisciplinarity of a field is also a factor which could affect a research group's tendency to collaborate. If the required knowledge cannot be found within one research group this has to be attained from external collaboration. Wagner (2005) categorised scientific research fields according to four motivation factors influencing collaboration: (1) data driven, (2) resource driven, (3) equipment driven, and (4) idea/theory driven. Data driven collaborations are defined as the incentive to share data with relevant partners. Access to data has become a major driver in health sciences in the attempt for larger clinical studies or access to data on different populations. Resource driven collaborations are often associated with unique and rare resources such as access to samples from individuals with rare diseases. Equipment driven collaboration implies cost-sharing, maintenance, and access to – but not necessarily sharing of – large-scale equipment. In the health sciences it could include access to advanced PET cameras or large magnetic resonance imaging machinery. Finally, idea/theory driven collaboration implies some kind of knowledge transfer and it is the driving factor every time the necessary knowledge required for a study is not covered by any of the researchers attached to the research group.

The Geographical Dimension

When examining the increase of co-authored articles in more detail it becomes obvious that international collaborations have increased more than domestic ones. In a period of more than 20 years (1988–2010), the ratio of international co-authored papers grew from 8 per cent of the world's total Science and Engineering articles to 24 per cent; the corresponding growth for national collaboration was 32 per cent to 43 per cent (National Science Foundation, 2012). Other studies have also observed this trend. In a study performed by Adams et al. (2005) it was observed that national collaboration between universities or universities and firms in the USA doubled between 1981 and 1999, while international collaboration over the same period increased five-fold. The pattern of increased international collaboration is more obvious in EU countries than in the USA. Japan and the average EU country have increased their international collaboration three-fold, while in the USA a two-fold increase could be observed (Archibugi and Coco, 2004).

Once again, differences exist in how researchers collaborate between fields. Archibugi and Coco (2004) found that earth- and space sciences, followed by physics and mathematics, are the fields that collaborate mostly internationally. Biology and biomedical research are other fields where international collaborations are prevalent. Concerning USA's international collaboration, astronomy, mathematics and statistics, and physics are the most international fields while agriculture, biology, and medicine are the least international. Life science is the field were international collaboration has increased the fastest (Adams et al., 2005). A questionnaire carried out with American institutions by Bozeman and Corley (Bozeman and Corley, 2004) showed that zoology, mathematics, materials engineering, and psychology were the most international fields while industrial engineering, mechanical engineering, health professions, biochemistry, and other biological and life sciences were the least collaborative.

In my earlier work (Mattsson et al., 2008) I made a distinction between intra-European (collaboration taking place only between researchers based in Europe) and extra-European collaboration (collaboration taking place between a European country and one or more partners from outside Europe). In the field of 'Clinical Medicine' (CM) (using the Science Citation Index definition) I found that collaboration with researchers based in the same country were most common. I also found that differences between countries exist, with researchers based in large European countries being more prone to collaborate nationally then researchers in small countries. The most likely explanation is that the choice of finding a suitable partner in a larger country with many researchers is higher than in a smaller country with a limited number of researchers with required knowledge. Therefore researchers in smaller countries have to look for appropriate partners outside the national borders. These differences only exist when observing collaboration with other European countries but are non-existing when studying co-publications between European and non-European countries. In the same article I investigated the frequency of multilateral collaboration involving researchers from at least three countries and found that Clinical Medicine was the field with the most countries included in the address fields of publications, with an average of 3.7 countries per article. Other fields investigated included Agriculture, Biology and Environmental Sciences (ABES); Clinical Medicine (CM); Life Sciences (LS); Physical, Chemical and Earth Sciences (PCES); Engineering and Computing and Technology (ECT).

The fact that geographical proximity, as well as cultural and language similarities between countries, have an impact on the way actors in different countries collaborate, has been observed by Zitt et al. (2000). Katz (1994) for example found that distance has a negative correlation on the collaboration frequency. If that is the case why do we then see this increasing trend in international co-authorship? Earlier studies have observed that co-publications receive more visibility measured by citations (Lewison and Cunningham, 1991; Rigby and Edler, 2005). Glänzel and Schubert (2001) and Persson et al. (2004) studied the subject in more detail and found that internationally co-authored publications have a higher citation rate than those resulting from domestic collaboration. Others have looked at the 'core' journals (most cited) of a specific field and found that the number of co-authored papers is higher than in other journals (Beaver and Rosen, 1978; Gordon, 1980). Research activity, as expressed by the number of publications of the individual author, has also been shown to increase, when collaborations are carried out (Persson et al., 2004), even though differences between scientific fields exist. It thus seems like the benefits that are associated with collaboration outweigh the disadvantages related to geographical distance.

Bibliometrics as a Method to Study Collaboration

Bibliometrics has been used in a wide range of different settings such as exploring the impact of a journal, paper or field. It is also more and more frequently used by policy makers for assessment purposes or by funding agencies as a tool to allocate funding to researchers (Adam, 2002). There are three types of bibliometric indicators: quantity indicators measuring the productivity of a particular research actor; quality indicators measuring the quality (also called performance) of an actor's output; and structural indicators measuring connections between publications, authors, and areas of research (Rehn and Kronman, 2008). In this chapter I focus on the latter by illustrating how co-publications can be used to study and measure structures and dynamics of scientific collaboration within the health science field.

The use of bibliometric indicators comes with both pros and cons. The argument for using co-authorship as an indicator of research collaboration is based on the fact that research results do not become acknowledged and recognised until the rest of the research community is aware of them. It is therefore essential for researchers to publish their results. If several researchers have contributed to the work that led to the results it is common practice, according to the Vancouver Group, that these should be included in the author list of the written work (ICMJE, 1997). Additionally, using bibliometrics as a method makes it possible to examine a large set of data, which is of particular importance when studying international collaboration. When using co-publications as an indication of collaboration it is important to keep in mind that some forms of collaboration do not result in co-published articles but may rather involve the sharing of research infrastructure, exchange of material or samples, intellectual property or some kind of informal collaboration which involve the stimulation of knowledge creation. Bibliometrically-supported comparisons between fields also need to be approached with caution. Differences may be due to different publication strategies. For example, mathematicians and other theorists tend to publish less than researchers in experimentally intensive fields such as in most of the sub-fields of Life Science (Moed et al., 2005) and health sciences. Similarly, publications in the field of physics do on average involve more authors than articles in the field of chemistry (Archibugi and Coco, 2004) due to the need to share large international infrastructure.

The data used for carrying out the analysis was retrieved from the Thomson Scientific (formerly Institute of Scientific Information) online database Web of Science (WoS). The WoS database is the most commonly used data source for

Table 2.1   Time span and number of articles included in the analysis

Time span	Total number of articles
1980–1982	9,250
1987–1989	10,537
1994–1996	15,216
2001–2003	18,203
2008–2010	19,078

carrying out bibliometric analysis even though it has a number of limitations (Moed, 2002) such as including only the largest and leading journals and having an Anglo-Saxon and American bias. The WoS database includes a number of different types of scientific documents such as book reviews, communications, conference abstracts, and letters. For the purpose of studying 'new science' only articles were selected for further analysis and reviews and other commentary or republication of already published materials were excluded.

Given the focus in this book on health sciences, it is important to provide a classification and a definition of this field. WoS has its own subject area classification of journals. In total there are 249 so called Category Terms. These Category Terms are clustered into five different Research Areas (Arts Humanities; Life Sciences Biomedicine; Physical Sciences; Social Sciences; Technology). For the purpose of this book the WoS classification Life Sciences Biomedicine is too broad. Therefore the OECD classification of WoS Category Terms was used instead. The OECD classification hierarchy is broken up into two levels: six major codes and 39 minor codes. The major codes are too broad as well, so the minor codes were selected instead. The minor codes 'Clinical Medicine' and 'Health Sciences' were selected for further analysis, since they best fit the focus of this volume. Each of these two minor codes then consists of a number of different Category Terms, mentioned above. For 'Clinical Medicine' there are 29 different Category Terms and for 'Health Sciences' there are 15 different Category Terms. Each of these different Category Terms includes a number of different scientific journals. The journal with the highest Impact Factor in each Category Term was selected for further analysis. To be able to analyse the evolvement of collaboration data all articles for each of the selected 41 journals were retrieved from five different time spans (1980–1982; 1987–1989; 1994–1996; 2001–2003; 2008–2010). In Table 2.1 the number of articles for each time span is presented.

The information found in the WoS database includes title of the article, language, names of authors, addresses of authors, journal information, reprint address (address of the corresponding author), and references. For the purpose of this chapter, information regarding author name and address(es), as well as references, were explored further and downloaded into a database.

Table 2.2   Statistics about authors

Time interval	Avg. # authors/paper	Median	Highest # authors
1980–1982	3.88	4	26
1987–1989	4.59	4	45
1994–1996	5.72	5	394
2001–2003	6.32	6	536
2008–2010	7.51	7	610

The Co-authorship Landscape in Health Sciences

In this section I present the results from the studies of co-authorship within the field of health sciences. More specifically, I analyse and discuss three different dimensions of collaboration within the field of health sciences. First, I present the structural properties of the co-publication networks including the number of authors and addresses and type of organisation. Second, I discuss the interdisciplinarity of health sciences through analysing references. Third, I investigate the geography of health science collaboration through the involvement of different countries.

First, I investigated the evolution of the size of the publication network by looking at the number of authors in each article. This was done by measuring the average number of authors per paper in all articles from the selected journals for each of the different time intervals (see Table 2.2).

The number of authors per paper has almost doubled over the last three decades from an average of 3.88 in 1980–1982 to 7.51 in 2008–2010. Also the median has increased from 4 authors per paper to 7 in 2008–2010. These results are in line with earlier research and confirm the trend of more authors being included in a publication. I further test the maximal number of authors that are involved in a publication. This indicator points towards an increasing collaboration rate. In 1980–1982, the publication with the largest number of authors included in a paper was 26 authors while the same number was 610 in 2008–2010. The number of publications that included more than both 50 and 100 authors was highest in 1994–1996. A closer look at the content of these publications indicates that they often involve some kind of randomised clinical trial involving patients in many different countries and/or hospitals. In 2001–2003 and 2008–2010 the number of papers with more than 50 and 100 authors declined. One explanation for this could be that a number of journals have introduced a policy that limit the number of authors to be included in a paper.

Next, I studied the number of different addresses mentioned in a publication and I observed the same pattern as for the number of authors involved in a paper. The average number of addresses has increased from 1.86 per paper in 1980–1982 to 4.27 in years 2008–2010. A similar increase can be observed when studying the median, see Table 2.3.

Table 2.3   Statistics about addresses

Time interval	Avg. # addresses/paper	Median	Largest # addresses
1980–1982	1.86	1	21
1987–1989	2.07	2	25
1994–1996	2.49	2	86
2001–2003	3.24	3	89
2008–2010	4.27	3	79

If we compare the number of authors included in a publication with the number of address we can conclude that the percentage of articles that have more addresses included than author names have increased (1980–1982, 35 per cent; 1987–1989, 18 per cent; 1994–1996, 16 per cent; 2001–2003, 30 per cent; 2008–2010, 35 per cent). This is an indication that authors are affiliated with more institutions or departments. Whether these can be considered as inter-institutional collaboration or not is discussed in Katz and Martin (1997). On the one hand only one single author is involved in the collaboration but at the same time a dual affiliation reflects some kind of an agreement between departments or institutions to share a researcher which could be considered a collaboration since knowledge is being actively shared.

Further analysis of the address fields can reveal collaboration between different sectors such as industry, academia, and hospitals. Here, I report a preliminary search for organisations that can be classified into these sectors to get an overview of the evolution of participation from different sectors. I investigated the addresses in detail to find out which organisations could be classified as a university, hospital/ clinic, or company. The participation of researchers from all sectors has increased due to increasing collaboration (more addresses in each article). Universities, to no surprise, are the most common type of organisation (~70 per cent in 1980–1982 and ~85 per cent in 2008–2010). The involvement of hospitals has also increased from ~35 per cent in 1980–1982 to ~45 per cent in 2008–2010. As for companies, the largest increase can be observed from ~1 per cent in 1980–1982 to ~6 per cent in 2008–2010. In addition different types of institutes, associations, government agencies, and centres are participating. The increasing involvement of different organisations from different sectors indicate that research in health sciences is becoming increasingly interdisciplinary and dependent on different types of knowledge but also an increasing dependency between the producers and users and a stronger link between bench to bedside.

Another method which can be used to study the interdisciplinarity of health sciences is to examine the references included in articles. As mentioned above, each journal included in the WoS database is classified into a subject field or Category Terms. Therefore each reference included in the articles can also be classified into a Category Term. In Figure 2.1 the results are presented in a graph for the five selected time periods.

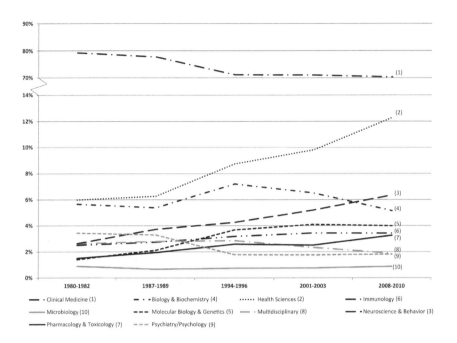

Figure 2.1   Evolution of references according to the 10 most common cited scientific fields

An overall observation is that the number of references included in a paper in Clinical Medicine and Health Sciences has increased from an average of 23 references per article in 1980–1982 to 38 references per article in 2008–2010. As expected the majority of references have been published in Clinical Medicine and Health Sciences classified journals. Still the number of references from other fields has increased over the years. The second most important source of knowledge comes from journals classified as 'Biology and Biochemisty' until 2008–2010 when 'Neuroscience and Behaviour' became more important. Also references classified in the area of 'Molecular Biology and Genetics' have increased. In general, I can conclude from this analysis that health sciences is relying on a growing number of knowledge sources as indicated by increasing number of references as well as references from different fields.

Third and final, I investigated the geographical dimension by studying the inclusion of authors from different countries in publications. An article was assigned to a country based on the information in the address field. Each link between distinctive countries was calculated maximally once per article. The number of countries that are involved in the knowledge production of health sciences has increased over the years studied. In the period 1980–1982 researchers from 97 countries published articles in journals classified as health

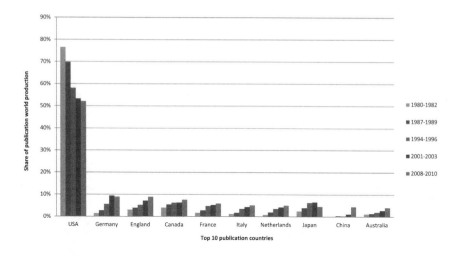

Figure 2.2   Share of the top 10 publication countries in the world production of health sciences publications

sciences. In 2008–2010 the number of different countries found in the address field was 162 (1987–1989, 107 countries; 1994–1996, 137 countries; 2001–2003, 142 countries). This result indicates that the field is becoming more international with researchers from many different countries participating in the knowledge generation.

Furthermore, I looked at the share of the total production of articles in health sciences for a subset of countries. Figure 2.2 illustrates the evolution of the top 10 countries producing articles in the health sciences field in 2008–2010.

The dominance of USA in the production of publications in the health sciences has been declining over the three decades studied, but US-based researchers still publish more than half (52 per cent) of all the articles in the field. The share of the other top nine producing countries in 2008–2010 has increased over time. The most interesting increase in number of published articles among top 10 countries can be seen in the case of China. In 1980–1982 researchers from China was on place 47 of publishing countries, only publishing six articles. In 2008–2010 China is the ninth most productive country with 893 articles.

Since we are interested in collaboration it is not enough to state that researchers based in more countries are participating in the knowledge production. We also want to investigate if more countries are participating in co-publications with other countries. One way of doing this is to study number of countries involved in each of the publications (or researchers from different countries represented in them).

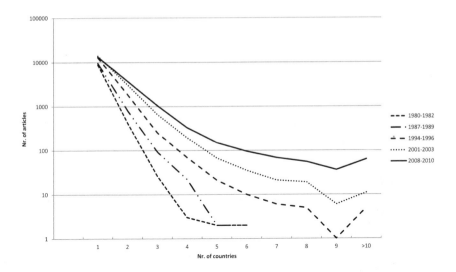

Figure 2.3   Number of articles with a specific number of countries in the address field

Figure 2.3 shows that the average number of countries in a publication has increased. In the time period 1980–1982 only one article included researchers from more than 10 countries in 2008–2010 that number increased to 63 (the highest number of countries in one article was 31).

Conclusion

In this chapter I presented findings from earlier literature on the evolution of collaboration, as well as novel results from bibliometric analyses of co-publications within health sciences. I focused on three different dimensions of collaboration: structural properties of the co-authorship network, interdisciplinarity and geographical dimensions in collaboration. In accordance with earlier literature I found that the amount of publications in the health sciences increased and co-publication increased even more. According to several studies, large differences exist between scientific fields and these have to be taken into account. After all, different fields are motivated by different needs in their search for appropriate collaborations, as well as by cultural differences.

The structure of the scientific networks has changed over the last decades both according to size and actors involved. According to earlier literature, the health sciences are the field that involves most authors in the publications after physics and astronomy where collaboration evolves around large scale infrastructures. Research in health sciences is often driven by the need to carry out clinical studies which relies on finding a relevant population, collection of samples, treatment of samples and their analysis. This is a time consuming process often involving many different people at different locations – hospitals and universities. In the analysis carried out in this chapter I found that the number of authors involved in a health science paper has doubled over the last three decades. The results with the highest number of authors in a publication summarise this trend: the number was more than 23 times larger in 2008–2010 compared to 1980–1982. Even though these large author networks have produced some ground breaking results, their emergence has also caused some problems for journals and institutions as highlighted by Kennedy (2003). The more serious problem presents itself when research misconduct is suspected. Questions asked by the author include 'should the liability be joint and several, accruing to all authors?' If not, then how should it be allocated among them? If there is an honest mistake in one part of the work but not in others, how should an evaluator aim his or her critique? Co-authors in these large networks rarely, or never, contribute equally to the work. As the interest in using bibliometric indicators for resource allocation and career development is getting more important in the process of understanding the individual author's contribution the above mentioned questions require more attention from authors, journals, as well as those distributing resources and deciding over careers. Such a discussion would also provide a constructive contribution to the meaning of co-authorship in the light of evaluating scientific careers, as well as in knowledge production in general.

The number of addresses mentioned in a paper increased as well as the percentage of articles that have more addresses included than author names. The last observation implies that authors have multiple affiliations. Similar patterns can be found in other fields but not to the same extension. The most likely explanation is the role of hospitals in health sciences. Access to clinical data and patients is a necessity for the research to be carried out. Many researchers split their time between clinical work and research and do therefore have an affiliation with both university or researcher institute and hospital or clinic. The analysis of addresses also indicated what types of organisations authors publishing in health sciences journals represent. It showed that in 1980–1982 the participation of authors from the industry was minor but since then the role of companies in research has become increasingly important.

As has been argued earlier in this chapter the interdisciplinarity of a research project influences the way researchers collaborate. If the knowledge required to answer a specific research question or to carry out a certain methodology is not available within one research group or department it might be necessary for a research group to search for that knowledge outside its own research field. In this chapter I used references to study the degree of interdisciplinarity among health sciences publications. The first observation was that the number of references per paper has increased, indicating that publications rely on an expanding knowledge pool. The majority of references can be found in the life science fields but the number of references to other fields such as social sciences, agriculture, physics, mathematics, or engineering has increased, implying that the health sciences are becoming more interdisciplinary. This does not differ from the general observation of science becoming more complex with the need of different subspecialties but rather confirms this trend.

The last dimension of collaboration I investigated in this chapter was the geographical evolution. This was done by studying the address fields and the countries where authors are based. To summarise, health sciences is becoming more international as indicated by the increasing number of researchers from different countries contributing to the knowledge production. This claim is supported by the increasing number of countries found in the address field in general but also by the increasing number of countries per publication. This increasing internationalisation is further supported by studying the share of total publications per country. The trend is that US is losing its position as the absolute dominant producer of health sciences in favour of other countries. Especially emerging countries are climbing the publication production list and I expect this trend to continue as their investment in research continues.

According to the literature review above, differences exist between scientific fields when it comes to the degree of internationalisation. The most international fields include astronomy and physics which is due to the international large scale infrastructures. Also mathematics is very international even though the number of authors in each publication is rather low in comparison. One possible explanation is the specific knowledge need in relation to the number of authors active in the field which might make it difficult to find a suitable collaboration partner within the national border. In an earlier study by Mattsson et al. (2008) clinical medicine (also included in this study) was found to be the least internationally collaborative field. At first sight this is surprising, since applied sciences, such as health sciences, are often more experimentally oriented and therefore come with a stronger need to collaborate (de Solla Price, 1963; Hagstrom, 1965; Gordon, 1980; Frame and Carpenter, 1979; Luukkonen et al., 1992). In addition, collaboration in this field can be motivated by the objective to share data related to for example statistics and clinical tests. However, the types of collaboration most suitable and practiced for researchers active in health sciences may unfold at the national rather than at the international level, since clinical trials, for example, can benefit from proximity. Therefore local or national collaboration between universities and hospital are often common. This is further supported by the finding that multiple affiliations, which are more likely to involve institutions in one and the same country, are most common among authors in clinical medicine classified publications. The role of ethical and legal differences between countries is also an aspect to take into account when explaining the propensity to collaborate with researchers outside national borders. National regulations on how human biological materials can be collected, stored, and used for certain purposes with respect for the personal integrity of the individual sometimes limit the exchange of material and data between countries e.g. the Swedish 'Biobanks in Health Care Act'. There are also differences in the way researchers collaborate in health sciences in different countries. For example, researchers in larger countries are more likely than those in smaller countries to collaborate with researchers based in the same country since the likelihood to find someone with the necessary knowledge, expertise or tools is higher because of a larger pool of researchers.

This chapter demonstrates how bibliometric indicators can be used to study collaboration in the field of health sciences. Using co-authorship provides a good overview of the evolution of the field, but to be able to further understand researchers' behaviour, intentions, and strategies, qualitative methods should be used as a complementary resource. The majority of other chapters in this book therefore provide excellent complements to the macro analysis provided in this chapter.

References

Adam, D. 2002. The counting house. *Nature*, 415(6873), 726–9.

Adams, J.D., et al. 2005. Scientific teams and institutional collaboration: Evidence from U.S. universities, 1981–1999. *Research Policy*, 34(3), 259–85.

Archibugi, D. and Coco, A. 2004. International partnerships for knowledge in business and academia – A comparison between Europe and the USA. *Technovation*, 24(7), 517–28.

de Beaver, D. and Rosen, R. 1978. Studies in scientific collaboration. *Scientometrics*, 1(1), 65–84, http://dx.doi.org/10.1007/BF02016840.

Bozeman, B. and Boardman, P.C. 2003. *Managing the New Multipurpose, Multidiscipline University Research Centers: Institutional Innovation in the Academic Community*.IBM Center for The Business Government.

Bozeman, B. and Corley, E. 2004. Scientists' collaboration strategies: Implications for scientific and technical human capital. *Research Policy*, 33(4), 599–616.

Frame, J.D. and Carpenter, M.P. 1979. International research collaboration. *Social Studies of Science*, 9(4), 481–97.

Glanzel, W. and Schubert, A. 2001. Double effort = double impact? A critical view at international co-authorship in chemistry. *Scientometrics*, 50(2), 199–214.

Gordon, M.D. 1980. A critical reassessment of inferred relations between multiple authorship, scientific collaboration, the production of papers and their acceptance for publication. *Scientometrics*, 2(3), 193–201.

Hagstrom, W.O. 1965. *The Scientific Community*. New York: Basic Books.

ICMJE 1997. Uniform requirements for manuscripts submitted to biomedical journals. *Journal of the American Medical Association*, 277, 927–34.

Katz, J.S. 1994. Geographical proximity and scientific collaboration. *Scientometrics*, 31(1), 31–43.

Lewison, G. and Cunningham, P. 1991. Bibliometric studies for the evaluation of trans-national research. *Scientometrics*, 21(2), 223–44.

Luukkonen, T., Persson, O. and Sivertsen, G. 1992. Understanding patterns of international scientific collaboration. *Science, Technology and Human Values*, 17(1), 101–26.

Mattsson, P., et al. 2008. Intra-EU vs. extra-EU scientific co-publication patterns in EU. *Scientometrics*, 75(3), 555–74.

Mattsson, P., et al. 2010. What do European research collaboration networks in life sciences look like? *Research Evaluation*, 19(5), 373–84.

Mattsson, P. 2012. Unpublished data.

Moed, H., Glänzel, W. and Schmoch, U. 2005. *Handbook of Quantitative Science. The Use of Publication and Patent Statistics in Studies of S and T Systems*. Dordrecht: Kluwer Academic Publishers.

National Science Foundation 2008. *Science and Engineering Indicators 2008*. http://www.nsf.gov/statistics/seind08/.

National Science Foundation 2012. *Science and Engineering Indicators 2012*. http://www.nsf.gov/statistics/seind12/.

Persson, O., Glanzel, W. and Danell, R. 2004. Inflationary bibliometric values: The role of scientific collaboration and the need for relative indicators in evaluative studies. *Scientometrics*, 60(3), 421–32.

Pritchard, A. 1969. Statistical bibliography of bibliometrics. *Journal of Documentation*, 25(4), 348–9.

Rehn, C. and Kronman, U. 2008. *Bibliometric Handbook for Karolinska Institutet*. Stockholm: Karolinska Institutet University Library.

Rigby, J. and Edler, J. 2005. Peering inside research networks: Some observations on the effect of the intensity of collaboration on the variability of research quality. *Research Policy*, 34(6), 784–94.

Smith, M. 1958. The trend toward multiple authorship in psychology. *American Psychologist*, 13, 596–9.

Swedish government 2002. *Biobanks in Health Care Act*, 2002, 297.

de Solla Price, D.J. 1963. *Little Science, Big Science*. New York: Columbia University Press.

Vermeulen, N., Parker, J.N. and Penders, B. 2013. Understanding life together: A brief history of collaboration in biology. *Endeavour*, 37(3), 162–71.

Zitt, M., Bassecoulard, E. and Okubo, Y. 2000. Shadows of the past in international cooperation: Collaboration profiles of the top five producers of science. *Scientometrics*, 47(3), 627–57.

PART II
Collaboration in Health Research

Chapter 3

From Virus to Vaccine: Projectification of Science in the VIRGO Consortium

Niki Vermeulen

After the Spanish flu in 1918 (40 million deaths estimated), the Asian flu in 1957 (40–50 per cent of the world population affected and about 2 million deaths), and the Hong Kong flu in 1968 (between 1 and 3 million deaths estimated), it has been assumed that another flu pandemic is likely, if not inevitable (Health Protection Agency, 2006; Kolata, 1999; Quammen, 2012; WHO, 2005a; 2005b). Risks are higher than ever, as within our modern society with its global transport infrastructure a virus that infects humans will spread even quicker than during previous pandemics (Bijker, 2006). This is why since the beginning of the new millennium, governments have been preparing for such a global outbreak, in collaboration with science and industry. In this context, the Netherlands Genomics Initiative funded an 'innovative project' combining academic and industrial research to develop a new vaccine against influenza: the VIRology GenOmics Consortium (VIRGO) that studies respiratory viral infections such as flu. While aiming to prevent another pandemic, this research project is also the embodiment of the increasing emphasis on innovation in research policy and the shaping of science as a manageable process, featuring strategies, roadmaps, and projects with acronyms and logos. As reflections on the meaning and impact of this 'projectification of science' are seldom found, this chapter will analyse the VIRGO collaboration as an example of projectification in health related research.

With important roots in traditional 'Big Science' projects like the Manhattan Project and the Apollo space programs, project design and management developed in fields of construction and engineering during the 1960s (Cicmil and Hodgson, 2006; Hodgson, 2004; Lock, 2003; Weinberg, 1969). As part of the New Public Management (Ferlie et al., 1996; Boston et al., 1996), the 1990s saw the project mode expanding across industries and other sectors, which is aptly described as the 'projectification of society' (Midler, 1995). Science has not escaped and has also become increasingly subject to projectification (Torka, 2006; Vermeulen, 2009). Collaboration predominantly takes place in a project format, which determines not only the structure of the research process but also influences the content of science.

In general, the propagation of the project mode of management is accompanied by a discourse on the project as an organisational response to the challenges of managing in a world of growing complexity (Cicmil and Hodgson, 2006; Hodgson, 2004; Lock, 2003; Midler, 1995; Sahlin-Anderson, 2002). The project's origin in modernity gives it a rational basis and a functionalist and instrumental view, focussing on time, cost, and output. But at the same time the project is presented and adopted as a new working mode in late- or post-modern societies that replaces the modern, hierarchical bureaucratic mode of organisation. Projects promise to deliver the ideal combination of a versatile and flexible but predictable form of work organisation, one that delivers controllability and adventure as well as decentralisation and accountability. However, more critical accounts on project management show that the world of projects is inhabited by dilemmas and contradictory logics. There is a gap between theory and practice and it is common knowledge that many projects cost more time and money than projected. Evaluation reports and studies provide insights in frequent cost overruns, substantial delays and under-performance. So while the project is widely adopted as an organisation format, its effectiveness as a management strategy is subject to discussion, now also extending into the realm of science.

What does the adoption of a project mode of working in scientific practice entail? Most obviously, the scientific project formalises scientific enquiry, via diverse forms of contracts: legal, financial, and technical. In addition, projects are a way of packaging inquiry more formally, through a design that considers a clearly defined problem that has a solution and a deliverable at the end. As the construction of a project proposal become the first step in doing research, the project mode of working adds an extra phase to scientific practice. Consequently, the discourse of 'the project' acts to mark out a specific time and space horizon within which the project is to be undertaken and evaluated. Thereby a separate, temporary organisational entity is created, with its own name, acronym, logo, and website, which sets it apart from other organisational entities like universities, research groups, and funding agencies. Each scientific project tells its own story; the project comes with the creation of a narrative constructed by people talking and writing about the project, for instance in project descriptions and proposals. This narrative legitimises the scientific project and contextualises it, by embedding it into broader narratives like discourses on scientific progress or societal problems. As a result, the projectification of science brings new roles for scientists, as they have to combine doing science with research management or the commercialisation of research.

This chapter further explores the projectification of science by analysing how in the VIRGO consortium the project format structures research. Based on qualitative research including document analysis and interviews, my analysis combines the triple-helix theory (Etzkowitz and Leydesdorff, 1998; 2000; Etzkowitz and Webster, 1998; Shinn, 2002) and the concept of boundary technology (Gieryn, 1983; 1995; 1999; Guston, 2001; Star and Griesemer, 1998) to get insight into the dynamics of the projectification of science: understanding the project as a 'boundary organisation' that enables the connection of government, academia, and industry. By presenting the VIRGO consortium, its construction and its organisation, this chapter will analyse the ways in which the project format influences research. I will argue that the project format serves as a tool to facilitate connections in the triple-helix, through organisational structure, control and accountability, time, space, and the career paths of scientists. However, my analysis of VIRGO also indicates some clear tensions between (biomedical) research and project work and shows how the logic of science is repeatedly compromised. This opens up questions on the appropriateness and innovativeness of this form of research organisation.

Making the VIRGO Consortium

In the context of the sudden spread of SARS and the thread of H5N1 and increasing attention to the risk of pandemics, scientists have been publicly propagating influenza research and the development of vaccines, while simultaneously unfolding a research agenda. For instance, Professor Ab Osterhaus, Head of the Department of Virology of the Erasmus Medical Centre in Rotterdam, frequently appeared in the Dutch media speaking of the risk of an influenza pandemic. In an expert interview he explained his position on the importance of virology research:

> We cannot already make a vaccine against the next "pandemic" because the virus continuously changes. We do not even know for sure that it will be H5. So, what in my view should happen now is to take for example, a H5 or H9 subtype, make a prototype – a candidate vaccine that is already adjuvated – and test it with humans. However, these are very expensive studies; we are talking about a multiplicity of ten million euros. Industry will not finance this of course, because those vaccines cannot be sold as it actually is technology development and a whole new infrastructure should be developed. However, this is something that should be done right now. When starting at the moment of the outbreak of the pandemic, a year is needed before proving the safety and efficacy of the vaccination and another half a year to produce the vaccine. That means that one and a half year has passed and experience teaches us that the pandemic is already gone by then. It has already passed around. So I definitely think that now is the time to experiment with prototypes of vaccines to prove which technologies should be used to make effective and safe pandemic vaccines.[1]

With this reasoning Osterhaus eloquently created a sense of urgency. He mobilises the future in the present (Van Lente, 1993; Brown et al., 2000) and also gives his view on who should take action. He clearly points out that research should be financed by government, as industry will not perform the necessary research

---

1 Video interview with Professor Ab Osterhaus on the website of *Erfocentrum* (the Dutch national knowledge and educational centre for heredity and medical biotechnology), 24 October 2005. Retrieved 29 October 2007, http://www.biomedisch.nl/film/vogelgriepvirus.php.

because there is nothing for them to gain yet. Osterhaus thereby touches on the complex relationship between science, government, and industry in innovation. In preparation for a possible pandemic, governments have to invest in public research, which eventually can lead to the development and commercial production of vaccinations or other forms of therapy by the pharmaceutical industry. This is reflected in the VIRGO project that started as an academic adventure but became a collaboration with industry stimulated by the government.

The Academic Start of the Project

On the website of the Netherlands Genomics Initiative[2] the VIRGO consortium has been presented as a so-called 'Innovative Cluster', which means concretely that the research is formulated in response to a question from industry and that industry takes the lead in the organisation of research (Folstar, 2002: 3). In the case of VIRGO, the leading company was ViroNovative BV. So when I decided to investigate the VIRGO project, I assumed that the main person behind the project would be someone from this company. However, it soon turned out that in order to get to know something about the consortium I needed to get in touch with coordinator Dr Arno Andeweg, an academic researcher who is based in the group of Osterhaus at Erasmus Medical Centre, which is part of Erasmus University in Rotterdam, a public facility. So while the coordination of VIRGO is presented as an industrial affair, it has a basis in academia.

As it turns out, the research proposal was actually an idea of Andeweg himself. He has a background in biology and already began to be interested in infectious diseases during his studies. In his PhD research he focused on the Human Immunodeficiency Virus (HIV) under supervision of Osterhaus. After his graduation in 1995 he kept in touch with Osterhaus while working at several other research institutes where he became interested in genomics research, the latest development in molecular biology. At the beginning of the 2000s he returned to the group of Osterhaus: 'That is when I wanted to start this research' (interview with Andeweg, 2005).[3] Osterhaus supported him when he envisioned integrating genomics research into the study of virus infections in order to learn more about the interaction between host and virus. As a result, VIRGO uses genomics techniques to investigate host-virus interactions to improve the rational design of vaccination and other intervention strategies for respiratory virus infections like influenza.

The basic idea behind vaccines is that they prevent virus infections by artificially bringing the host into contact with the virus and teaching the host how to react without becoming ill. However, vaccines can either produce the good learning reaction or the unwanted reaction, so the crux is to know what makes the good reaction. However, until now the reaction is often a surprise:

---

2   Retrieved 29 October 2007, http://www.genomics.nl.

3   Interview with Dr Arno Andeweg, Coordinator of VIRGO, Department of Virology, Erasmus Medical Centrum, Rotterdam, the Netherlands, 29 April 2005.

We now basically do not have enough knowledge about the immune response of the host in case of a virus infection. So vaccine development is still largely depending on a "trial and error" approach. If an experimental vaccine works we have a new vaccine, but if it does not work we have to try something else again. (interview with Andeweg, 2005)

Genomics research can contribute to the understanding of the host response to a virus:

With the new genomics tools you can at every moment – this is like the time-axe within the black-box – and at each stage see which genes are turned on and which are turned off. With the new tools you now have the ability to look with a very high resolution into what exactly happens within the host and what happens if you change something in the virus or in the vaccine. (*Idem*)

This type of research gives better insight into the reaction of the host and can eventually rationalise the design of vaccines.

The new research approach had a slow start as Andeweg first had to work on ongoing projects, and only had little time to work on his own ideas. Only when a European project was granted, he secured part of it to start his own research, albeit on a small scale. However, soon he realised he needed a large-scale approach:

Genomics is big and technology development goes fast, so you actually cannot do this on a small-scale. This means that you need to realise, and this is my experience, that with only little money and little manpower you are always behind. And although it has your interest and it has potential, you will not be able to follow. (*Idem*)

Consequently, he tried to build a collaboration and to acquire more money. First, he became part of a larger effort within the Erasmus Centre to become a 'Centre of Excellence' specialising in infectious diseases within the then newly established Netherlands Genomics Initiative (NGI). Unfortunately, the proposal was not selected due to a lack of focus: 'That was not very surprising because they involved more and more groups to fulfil the requirement of a very large multi-disciplinary centre. Everything may seem fit in the end, but if you do not take care, you lose your focus' (*idem*). When the NGI came with a new call for research proposals Andeweg decided to give it another go and wrote his own proposal. However, the research proposal needed to be aligned with the goals and requirements of the call of the NGI.

The Netherlands Genomics Initiative

The VIRGO consortium is one of the projects of the Netherlands Genomics Initiative (NGI), a special agency within the general Netherlands Organisation for Research

Funding that was set-up in response to the 'genomics revolution' and developments in biotechnology. Following the lobbying of scientists and policymakers and the advice of a special committee, a political debate concluded that the Netherlands' genomics infrastructure was in need of a 'substantial reinforcement' (NGI, 2001).[4] With the support of five Dutch ministries – involved with, respectively, education and research, health, economic affairs, agriculture, and the environment – the NGI was founded in 2001 with a budget of €188.8 million to stimulate and coordinate the genomics knowledge infrastructure in the Netherlands.

The first activity of the NGI was the creation of a strategic plan (2002–2006):

> The Netherlands Genomics Initiative heads the decision-making process for the selection and stimulation of both existing and new research activities. It primarily supports an integrated approach, from fundamental research up to and including ultimate application and attention to societal aspects. Significant emphasis is also placed on the education of young people and the positioning of genomics in social, national and international spheres. (NGI, 2001: 3)

The strategy revolved around the word 'focus': on excellency, on social awareness and accountability, and on innovative potential. It was put into practice via an integrative approach consisting of 12 lines of action, most importantly the creation of 'Genomics Centres of Excellence' dedicated to fundamental research.

The creation of 'Innovative Clusters' only took place later, after the establishment of the Centres of Excellence. 'The idea of the creation of Innovative Clusters emerged within the Initiative itself, because in the Centres of Excellence industrial participation was missing' (interview with De Geus, 2005). Since the commercialisation of research was experienced as a difficult process, the NGI developed a valorisation policy to realise innovation in the life sciences, and the Innovative Clusters formed an important part of this policy. By explicitly giving industry the lead in research, the Innovative Clusters are the materialisation of new insights in innovation theory that picture innovation as a cyclical process, instead of a linear development from academia to industry (Berkhout, 2002). The Innovative Clusters were not financed by the NGI, but from BSIK funds – a funding programme that supports the transition towards a knowledge economy with revenues from the old economy: the exploitation of natural gas.[5] Under supervision of the NGI, seven proposals devoted to the life sciences were prepared and submitted to the BSIK programme. Of this so-called 'NGI omnibus proposal' six proposals were successful – amongst others the VIRGO consortium – and they were granted a total of €86 million of the BSIK funds.

---

4   In 2001 the Wijffels Committee produced the report on 'knowledge infrastructure genomics', commissioned by the Ministry of Education, Culture and Science.

5   BSIK is an abbrevation of 'Besluit Subsidie Investeringen Kennisinfrastructuur' which translates into 'Decision Funding Investment Knowledge Infrastructure'. Retrieved 2 November 2007, http://www.senternovem.nl/bsik/algemeen/-index.asp.

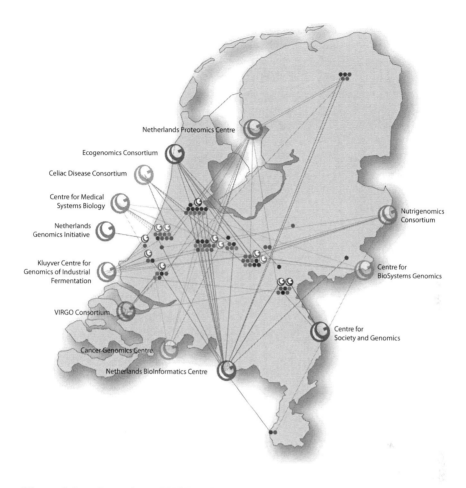

Figure 3.1   Overview of NGI activities in 2004

Source: Image courtesy of Netherlands Genomics Initiative (NGI, 2005b).

While the NGI was originally established for a period of five years, efforts to prolong the initiative with another five years started towards the end of this period. In the first five years the NGI has built a network of genomics research in the Netherlands:

> We have been able to make some changes. Parties are starting to organise themselves, take their responsibilities and this can only be understood as the result of our actions [...] We have effectively stirred things up. (Interview with De Geus, 2005)[6]

---

6   Interview with Dr Bernard de Geus, Project Coordinator, Netherlands Genomics Initiative, The Hague, the Netherlands, 16 March 2005.

This view was confirmed by an international panel of experts during the mid-term review, which also brought the issue of continuity to the fore: 'The panel was impressed by what has been achieved, but also expressed the view that more work will be required to achieve the desired and intended objectives' (NGI, 2006: 32). Based on an overview of results over the period 2002–2007 and a new strategy for the period 2008–2012 supported by industry (NGI, 2005a; 2005c; 2005d), the Dutch government decided in September 2007 to award the NGI €271 million for a second phase (NGI, 2007a). In these last years the NGI has concentrate especially on maximising the economic and societal value of the research as presented in the NGI Business Plan called 'Munt uit Genomics', which translates as 'Capitalising on Genomics' (NGI, 2007b).

Building an 'Innovative Cluster'

The Netherlands Genomics Initiative has played a crucial role in the building of VIRGO. After the decline of the first Rotterdam proposal for an NGI Center of Excellence in which Andeweg and his research would have had a place, Andeweg decided to try it with the support of Ab Osterhaus when the NGI came with the new call for proposals for the Innovative Clusters: 'it gave me the space to do what I was convinced of together with Osterhaus as a motivating factor' (interview with Andeweg, 2005). Working on the research plan took much time, and included discontinuing experimental work and working weekends:

> Setting up a research project is a big investment for a researcher and a research group, so you have to be able to find the time to actually participate in the competitions that enable you to scale-up your research. Personally, I created that time by more or less putting my experimental work on halt when my lab-analyst went on maternity leave. So I did not have to be in the lab that often and I could dedicate myself entirely to the research proposal. (*Idem*)

Based on previous experience, Andeweg made sure he kept his plans focused and therefore decided to concentrate only on respiratory viruses: the influenza virus, the Respiratory Syncytial Virus (RSV) and the human MetaPneumoVirus (hMPV). These targeted viruses are different enough to provide the necessary variety, while also being related. In addition, Andeweg did not organise meetings with collaborators during the writing process, but mainly communicated via email or bi-lateral meetings. Only after designing the research proposal were other research groups selected to be part of the research project.

Moreover, Andeweg had become well aware of the importance of the presentation of the project and he made the proposal readable and attractive for the evaluators. He made sure, for instance, to include diagrams in the research proposal.

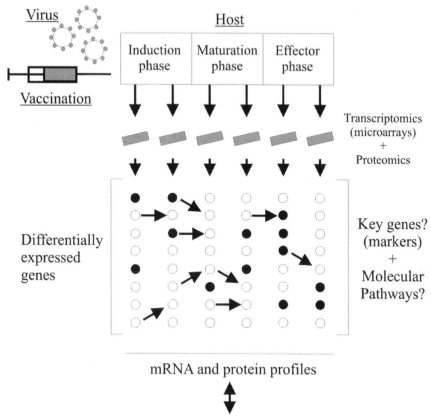

Figure 3.2   The schematic presentation of the application of genomics tools in research on the virus-host interaction

Source: Image courtesy of Arno Andeweg, VIRGO.

> I learned from the EU project in which I participated that they like pictures. This is simply what works and it is not artificial as I also like to think along these lines. When people have to read lots of this kind of paperwork [he flips through the elaborated research proposal], then it is important that you show with nice diagrams how the structure is built. (Interview with Andeweg, 2005)

Finally, Andeweg and Osterhaus baptised the collaboration VIRGO: a contraction of virology and genomics which also indicates that the research has not been done earlier.

In February 2003 the VIRGO research proposal was submitted and in the following months reviewed by several organisations:

From February till the summer numerous organisations have taken a look at it, from the Netherlands Bureau for Economic Policy Analysis to the National Institute for Public Health and the Environment and SenterNovem for economic-societal factors and of course the purely scientific review as well. (*Idem*)

The VIRGO team had to present the proposal four times in a row to different organisations, but it was worth the trouble. In November 2003 their efforts were rewarded with a grant of €10.8 million (NGI, 2003: 11).

But what about the participation of industry? When asking Andeweg about this, he acknowledged that the requirements for VIRGO were quite different from the requirements of the academic Centres of Excellence of the NGI. Most importantly, industry needs to be the leading party in an Innovative Cluster. Consequently, the VIRGO consortium put forward ViroNovative, a company that is dedicated to the human MetaPneumoVirus (hMPV) which was discovered by Osterhaus's group in 2001. This discovery resulted in the establishment of a new company that is located in the same building as Osterhaus's group, only two floors higher:

> This company is a spin-off of our group. So that was easy, as Ab [Osterhaus] is the scientific director of the company. We could perfectly combine the two so as to find a good solution. And we all work both above and here below anyway. This good "internal" public–private collaboration, then, provided the foundation for the expansion of public–private collaboration in the innovative cluster. (Interview with Andeweg, 2005)

According to Andeweg, the NGI knew that ViroNovative was not really the leading party behind the consortium, but this was not a problem as VIRGO is one of the clusters with most commercial ties.

Industrial involvement in VIRGO has indeed taken shape but only after the academic start of the project. This means that industry was not involved in the formulation of the question – as required by NGI – but Andeweg says about this:

> It depends on how you define what a question is. Pharma in general and Solvay [one of the participating companies] in particular, have a great interest in better vaccines, so there is a demand. It is only that they did not ask us explicitly to do this using genomics tools. (*Idem*)

Nevertheless, industrial parties became seriously involved in the research collaboration and contributed €3.3 million to the project (Boekholt et al., 2007). The industrial partners had different aims: ViroNovative wanted to exploit its IP position further by developing knowledge for marketable products for hMPV intervention strategies while Solvay Pharmaceuticals was interested in the development of knowledge for a new generation of human influenza vaccines. Next to ViroNovative and Solvay, Intervet took part in the project aiming to develop knowledge for animal vaccinations. The different orientations of the companies involved enabled them to build on the same knowledge without competing with each other.

Academic and industrial partners also agreed on being complementary. The academic partners remained to have primarily academic goals: the development of new knowledge about host-virus interaction on which future research can be build. However, coordinator Andeweg also acknowledged the importance of academia and industry working together, as it is important that academic research on vaccines has an outlet to companies. Moreover, the group of Osterhaus has a long-term tradition of cooperation with industry to supplement governmental research funding which is 'not always abundant'. The other way around, vaccine companies depend on public research as they are often not able to perform fundamental research themselves. The industrial partners therefore hope to acquire new fundamental knowledge through academic projects that can be further developed into marketable products. Jeroen Medema from Solvay Pharmaceuticals explains how VIRGO contributes to vaccine development:

> The VIRGO consortium is of great importance for vaccine producers. First of all, we do not have the capacity to carry out that kind of fundamental research ourselves. Our strategy is to monitor what is going on in universities and elsewhere and then jump on the bandwagon, preferably before it accumulated speed. That means we try and pick up new concepts at an early stage and develop them further through clinical trials, registration and market introduction. We expect VIRGO to feed our pipeline of new vaccines and medicines. (Medema cited in NGI, 2005e)

This quote confirms the importance of the collaboration for industry. Medema especially expected to use the VIRGO research to improve vaccines and reduce the time that is needed to develop a vaccine.

In short, the analysis of the formation of VIRGO shows how the research project is actually an academic collaboration that turned into a public–private collaboration led by a company due to the requirements of funding policy. The result was the VIRGO project proposal in which actors brought their different goals in line by combining fundamental research with industrial goals for application.

Organising the VIRGO Consortium

In the case of VIRGO the organisational structure of the project makes visible how academia, government, and industry have become entangled. First of all, the project has been connected to the Dutch government via its funding sources: the Netherlands Genomic Initiative and the BSIK funding programme, a collaboration between six Dutch government departments, including the Ministry of Education, Culture and Science which is responsible for the Innovative Clusters of the NGI. However, the monitoring of the BSIK programmes was delegated to SenterNovem,

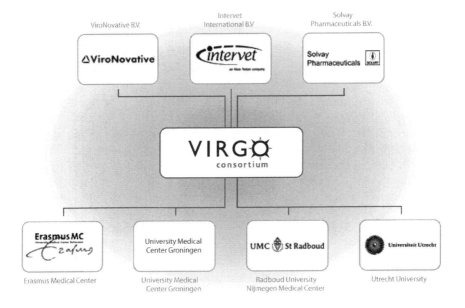

Figure 3.3   Partners in the VIRGO consortium

Source: Image courtesy of Arno Andeweg, VIRGO.

an agency of the Dutch Ministry of Economics Affairs that stimulates innovation. As a result the VIRGO consortium has been officially tied to two funding programmes and three government organisations. Moreover, the requirements of the funding organisations have connected the academic partners to the industrial partners in the collaboration.

The Project as a Triple-helix

The VIRGO consortium consists of research groups from four universities and three pharmaceutical companies. Next to the spin-off company ViroNovative (that has now become part of the American company MedImmune), Solvay Pharmaceuticals has been a long-term partner of the virology department in Rotterdam regarding research into human influenza and Intervet, specialising in animal pharmaceuticals, was already involved in genomics research, notably related to poultry. The academic partners involved in VIRGO are colleagues of Andeweg dispersed over four Dutch universities, specialising in virology, theoretical biology, medical microbiology, veterinarian medicine, pulmonary medicine, immunology, paediatrics, neurology, and bioinformatics. As all partners were already connected to the group of Osterhaus in some way, the VIRGO project solidifies already existing connections in its organogram.

Within this organisational structure, the research was divided into 10 so-called 'Work Packages': 'Of each WP we elaborated on the participants, the goals, the approach, the detailed approach, the milestones and the responsibilities' (interview with Andeweg, 2005). Each Work Package performed a specific part of the overall research plan and studied, respectively: host-virus interactions in target cells (1); mouse models (2); non-human primates (3); chickens (4); and humans (5) (Johnston et al., 2007). Other packages were dedicated to vaccine research (6); transcriptomics (7); proteomics (8); data storage, analysis, and mining (9); and the modelling of immune gene-interacting networks (10).

While the Work Packages were performing the research independently and each has its own research leader, they were related to each other through the overall aims of the research and the fact that they also build upon each other's work. For instance, the cell and animal studies were performed to find basic mechanisms of host-virus interaction that may also take place in humans. Therefore, Work Package 3, which uses non-human primates for experimentation, explicitly built on the work within WP 1, 2, and 4 in which respectively cells, mice and chickens were used as a model. WP 6, which performed research on vaccination, again built on WPs 1 to 4. In addition, WP 7 has been dedicated to technology development and standardisation for all projects and partners in the consortium, which is crucial for making data compatible. Finally, WP 9 and 10 integrated the data from all the other research efforts and built models.

Next to the individual management of the Work Packages, an overall management structure of the VIRGO consortium was set in place, consisting of a governing board, a general assembly and a steering board. The governing board reported to Senter and the NGI, while in the general assembly decisions about the project were taken. Each WP had a representative in the general assembly who represented one of the participating institutions at the same time. The steering board, in turn, was responsible for daily business. It was formed by Andeweg (as coordinator) in dialogue with Osterhaus (as official head of the project) and supported by a half-time secretary while some people with business experience were involved too. In addition, the project made use of the experience of an officer of the Technology Transfer Office of Erasmus MC to allocate IPR. Finally, legal and financial matters were outsourced to experts, respectively to the legal service of Erasmus MC and an outside accountancy firm.

VIRGO thus shows how the different domains of government, academia and industry have been tied together in an organisational structure of various layers. First of all, the core of the VIRGO consortium consists of academic and industrial research groups. Around this centre, government agencies are in place, as well as financial and legal support. Secondly, the project itself has various organisational levels. While at first sight the 14 different research groups all seem to collaborate, it turns out that the research is actually divided into 10 Work Packages in which specific groups work together. These groups are connected through the research results and via the management of the project. It is only on the management level that actors from all the different organisations come together. This structure binds the different domains together in a new organisational entity that forms the backbone of the research: the VIRGO project that enables the different societal orderings to connect and overlap.

Control and Accountability

Next to structuring the research and its governance, the project format deals with control and accountability of science. When talking to scientists in charge of a research project, you can be sure that they get started on 'bureaucracy' at some point, a term that scientists use to cover the things they certainly do not like: policy procedures and the pile of paperwork that comes with it. Originally bureaucracy does not have a negative connotation and it can also be argued that bureaucracy is the protector of freedom in scientific collaboration as it defines the participants' rights concerning data (Shrum et al., 2007). And although it is nowadays very much part of a career in science, for scientists, bureaucracy is often a major cause of frustration and the direct enemy of valuable research time (Parker et al., 2011). In this respect Andeweg is exemplary as he prefers government just handing out a bag of money without restrictions:

> Sometimes I wonder what happens if you just give researchers money and a direction of research and let them do their job. Of course things will go wrong, but the question is whether more things will go wrong? At least it would mean that more money is spent on research as now the costs for the whole apparatus are quite substantial, not only at the policy side, but also at the academic side. (Interview with Andeweg, 2005)

In this light, the need for an NGI was even questioned by scientists. For instance, the prominent Professor Piet Borst, former director of the Netherlands Cancer Institute, claimed:

> Already before the establishment of the NGI, excellent research in genomics was performed in the Netherlands. Researchers only needed money to be able to perform world-class research, but they did not need orchestration. They know themselves which research directions are promising. They needed help, not interference or extra bureaucracy. (Borst, 2004: 46)

From a scientific perspective the new NGI initiative with its elaborate strategies, fancy brochures and network meetings seems a waste of money, because it is the research that counts and that is where the money has to go.

A different perspective, however, also shows a different world. From a policy perspective De Geus from NGI states that the regulations and paperwork that come with the funding of science are simply essential:

The Netherlands Genomics Initiative is viewed as quite bureaucratic indeed, but this is all but true. Yes, we do have some rules people have to adhere to. But when we ask for reports of progress we want to know only about the general progress, not the details. Rather than lengthy reports of progress, we want concise ones. Accountability is the real problem, however. People just don't like to be accountable, especially scientists. But accountability is not a strange thing to ask for. When I award a research grant of some 16 million [Euro], I would think I'm entitled to know what happens with the money. [...] We are talking about public money here that should be accounted for. (Interview with De Geus, 2005)

On a European level, Dr Jacques Remacle, who is working for the part of the Directorate General for research that specialises in functional genomics, adds that the need for accountability increases together with the scale of research:

When dividing money over small research projects, it does not matter if one project does not deliver as the others will. However, when investing huge amounts of money in large research networks I need to know how the money is spent. (Interview with Remacle, 2005)[7]

Moreover, it is argued that research policy takes place on a playing field in which science is not the only player, and that research has to compete with other national and European priorities and should therefore produce tangible economic or social benefits in order to be legitimate.

These dissimilar scientific and policy perspectives on bureaucracy are to some extent reconciled in the VIRGO project. The project structure enabled the scientists to develop their own internal management practices, while also staying accountable to the funding organisation. On the one hand, the internal coordination of the project could be organised by participating scientists themselves, minimising bureaucracy. Within the VIRGO project they explicitly tried to keep the organisational structure simple:

In other consortiums they put an extra management layer in between, but they often take the bureaucracy of The Hague [the seat of government and many funding organisations] into the research projects [...] In contrast, we are very decisive compared to the sister projects who often have about three people being responsible for daily business. (Interview with Andeweg, 2005)

Initially, they chose Andeweg as the central coordinator: like a spider-in-the-web involved in research as well as management and communication towards outside organisations. And although participants sometimes got annoyed when Andeweg sent them too many different emails, they certainly appreciated the lack of

---

7   Interview with Dr Jacques Remacle, Policy Officer Unit F4, DG Research, European Commision, Brussels, Belgium, 6 October 2006.

bureaucracy. Nevertheless, during the course of the project they had to expand the management of the project by hiring a special project manager (personal communication with Andeweg, 2009).

On the other hand, the project format enables accountability and evaluation of science by making science open to external control. By constructing VIRGO as a research project, it becomes a separate organisational entity with pre-set goals that can be evaluated, not only at the beginning and the end of projects, but also at regular intervals in between. More concretely, in case of VIRGO three different evaluation procedures were in place. First, VIRGO started with a so-called 'zero measurement' in which the situation at the beginning of the project was pictured, followed by monitoring halfway and at the end. Secondly, reports of progress for the Netherlands Genomics Initiative had to be made every six months. In addition, VIRGO is part of evaluations of the NGI as a whole. Moreover, reports of progress not only focus on scientific results but also on the management process and societal evaluation criteria. As under the influence of government and industry standards of evaluation have become more diverse in comparison to the peer-review that is the common form of evaluation in the scientific domain. Therefore, evaluations also pay attention to the commercialisation of research results, such as the number of partners, patents and start-up companies.

Making Time and Space

Next to dealing with control and accountability, the project enables the creation of its own time and space. Firstly, the project intermediates between the different time regimes in science, government and industry. While research results can take quite some time and certainly do not come at a pre-set time, administrative time has an annual rhythm and is relatively short-term. Finally, industrial time is configured as 'time to market' (TTM), which refers to the time it takes to transform knowledge into a product that can be sold and which is ideally as short as possible. By going beyond these different orderings, the research project makes its own time. This coordination of different temporal regimes can be clearly seen at the start of VIRGO project. While the development of the new line of research by Andeweg already started at the end of the last century, the project proposal for VIRGO was handed in at the beginning of 2003. Although they soon heard that chances of funding were high, and funding was officially confirmed in October 2003, the year 2004 was well under way before they could officially start the research:

> In the summer [of 2003] we already knew that we were in second position concerning the science review of about 70 projects that would eventually get funded, so we knew we had a very big chance. But it took almost a year before we actually got the letter that we could start. That was around March or April 2004. And to make matters worse, we had to start retro-actively in January. (Interview with Andeweg, 2005)

So while the research project could only start after they received the letter, the official starting point of the project became the beginning of a new (administrative) year: January 2004.

Although the project format enables harmonisation of different timeframes through the creation of a project timeline, it proves difficult to connect them smoothly. This can not only be seen in the process of designating a common starting point, but also in the evaluation procedures. Although January 2004 was considered to be the project's starting point the research had not actually started yet, which turned the first six-month progress report into a problem because no research had taken place yet. A similar problem became apparent during the external evaluation of the Netherlands Genomics Institute in 2006. Four years after the start of the NGI, the initiative was subject to thorough evaluation, including the 11 research centres that were established under its supervision. As a result, also the VIRGO consortium was evaluated by an international review committee chaired by Sebastian Johnston, Professor of Respiratory Medicine at Imperial College in London. And although overall the consortium was evaluated as 'very good to excellent' the report stated:

> This evaluation is carried out prematurely as the Consortium only received confirmation of its funding in October 2004 and many of the Work Packages only started their work between 1 year and 1½ years ago. The Committee were really only able to review planned activities and preliminary data. Productivity for all Work Packages was impossible to assess. The scoring of the various Work Packages has potential to be considerably higher than that awarded in this assessment as there was little in the way of outputs available for review. The "Work in Progress" was generally considered to be of excellent quality. (Johnston et al., 2007: 11)

So Professor Johnston and his colleagues came all the way from the United Kingdom, Canada, Northern Ireland, and Spain while the time was not right.

In addition to time, different spatial orderings need to be aligned. While science and flu research is an international activity and also industry is often multi-national operating on global markets, government has a national orientation. Within the VIRGO project these different spatial orderings are realigned into a national space: it consists only of Dutch research institutes and companies located in the Netherlands. The funding source is the reason that VIRGO has become a national collaboration, as the NGI has been established to build a genomics research infrastructure within the Netherlands and does not support scientists from other countries and BSIK funding also has a national label. This tension between international and national also becomes apparent when analysing the output of VIRGO, which shows how publications were still predominantly international, while national publications show increasing collaboration between the consortium partners (Hessels et al., 2012; Hessels and Deuten, 2012).

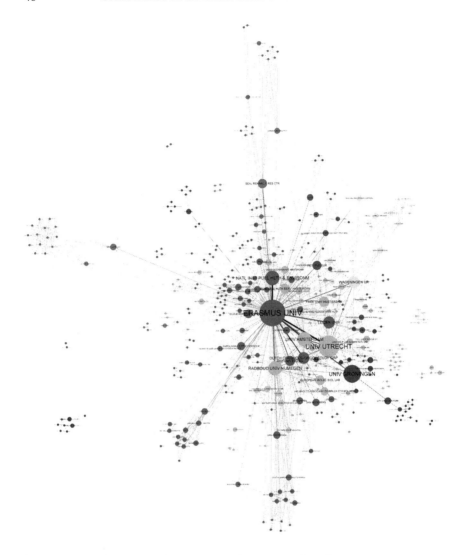

Figure 3.4   Map of publications showing connections between participating organisations from VIRGO in the period 2000–2003[8]

Only when the NGI later broadened its scope to include internationalisation as an objective, the international context of the VIRGO project became more acknowledged. As a result, the creation of VIRGO shows how sometimes a specific

---

8   With a special thank you to Edwin Horlings of the Rathenau Institute in The Hague for making this map, and CWTS, Leiden for providing part of the data.

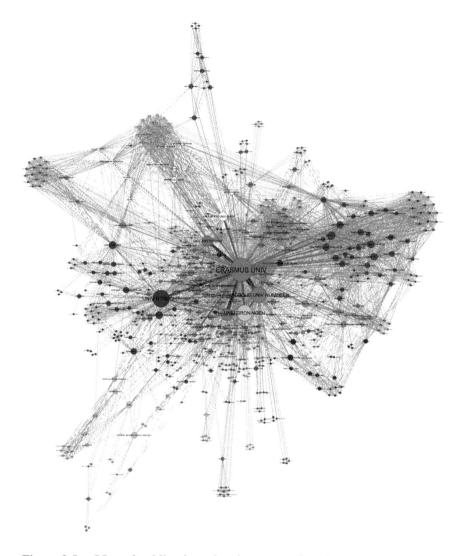

Figure 3.5   Map of publications showing connections between participating organisations from VIRGO in the period 2007–2010[9]

ordering can be more dominant in the new project configuration then others and the government proved to have the upper hand within VIRGO.

***

9   *Idem.*

New Roles for Scientists

When reflecting on his own role in the construction of VIRGO, Andeweg notes that building collaboration is a different way of doing science, as coordination and management become more important: 'The motivation to start such a project is the fascination for the content of the research, but in practice you gradually transform into a manager' (interview with Andeweg, 2005). Managing research can have important consequences for the career of a scientist. Building a new research project simply affects the academic performance of a scientist, as no time is left for performing research and writing publications:

> I just got to the point in this research project where I can start thinking of publishing again, but I didn't have that for years. Of course it does matter if you manage to acquire such a project, because it allows you to stay on a bit longer. But I made an enormous time investment that might as well have left me with nothing if the project would not have been funded. It is victory or death. (Interview with Andeweg, 2005)

In addition to the lure of management, the crossing of the boundary between academia and industry has implications on an individual level as well. For instance, within the Industrial Cluster format of VIRGO it would have been easier if Andeweg as the person in charge had started to work for the leading company ViroNovative. However, he explicitly refused to make the transfer to industry as he prefers being an academic:

> I simply do not want that. You will get the most bizarre situations, for it is all about money there, and you are also dependent on the decisions of the American parent company [...] My heart is with research and I want to do that within academia because I want to be independent. (*Idem*)

At the same time Andeweg states that being an academic increasingly can be compared to being an entrepreneur. Scientists can only perform research when they write research proposals. If in this case Andeweg made a clear choice to stay within academia, his role as an academic transformed anyway. He is forced to balance managerial interests and scientific standards: a double role.

Although Andeweg stays put, individual border crossings have become quite common within the scientific world these days (Shapin, 2008). Some scientists even seem to be particularly good at it: they manage to strike a balance between science, business and policy interests and in addition sometimes even master public communication. A famous example is Craig Venter who, after the beginning of his scientific career within the National Institutes of Health, reinvented himself as an entrepreneur competing with the public project to sequence the human genome and then became a non-profit scientist again (Shreeve, 2004; Venter, 2007). If this made him world famous, it also turned him into a scientist who is able to combine different roles, as is expressed by the well-known picture that shows Venter half as a scientists and half as a businessman. The official leader of VIRGO, Professor Ab Osterhaus, performs a similar hybrid role within the Dutch national context and the international community of influenza experts. He combines his role as a successful academic, with his roles as director of the Dutch National Influenza Centre, government advisor and entrepreneur. In addition, he regularly appears as an expert in all kinds of media to talk about the risks of influenza.

Although Osterhaus's embodiment of different identities has been an asset for the promotion of VIRGO in the different domains, the combination of different roles can also give rise to criticism. In the case of Osterhaus it was the epidemiologist Dr Luc Bonneux from the Belgium Health Care Centrum who took a stance against virologists who are predicting the coming of a pandemic and are at the same time advising governments to buy anti-viral medicines while also having ties to the pharmaceutical industry (De Rijck, 2005).[10] Consequently, Bonneux questions whether it is possible to combine the different identities in a single person, suggesting that a scientist should keep to their scientific role.

VIRGO Continued

While projects have a clear end, the research process continues to develop, providing new challenges and opportunities. Although the VIRGO project was granted for the period of 2004–2009 with a project extension till 2010, the participants were eager to continue the line of research that grew out of the combination of virology and genomics: 'We have learned from VIRGO and other scientific developments and we would like to broaden our ability and skills' (interview with Andeweg, 2012).[11] As the NGI was granted another five years after its initial period from 2002–2007, some NGI projects were refunded and this also provided opportunities for VIRGO. Despite good outcomes (over 200 peer reviewed publications and about 20 patent applications and licences) and evaluations of the initial VIRGO project, this did not lead to a continuation of NGI funding. NGI did not give a full second grant but a partial one to enable some continuation of the research and find additional funding which was provided by the Dutch Life Sciences Health sector

---

10   This critique was first formulated in a newspaper article in the Belgium national newspaper *De Standaard* and was followed by an interview on Dutch radio in 'De Ochtenden' on 19 October 2005, retrieved 1 December 2005, http://www.ochtenden.nl/afleveringen/23986305/, and a debate between Bonneux and Osterhaus on *NOVA*, a Dutch current affairs television programme, on 22 October 2005, retrieved 1 December 2005, http://www.novatv.nl/index.cfm?LN=nl&FUSEACTION=videoaudio.details&REPORTAGE_ID=3808.

11   Interview with Dr Arno Andeweg, Managing Director of VIRGO, Viroscience Lab, Erasmus Medical Centrum, Rotterdam, the Netherlands, Utrecht, 14 November 2012.

FES grant.[12] As a result, VIRGO II combines two funding sources thereby not only increasing the total research budget to about €30 million (including 50 per cent matching by the partners), but also the scale and scope of the project.[13]

VIRGO II explicitly builds on the work of VIRGO but the project has broadened in various ways. First of all, the single focus on acute, respiratory viruses has expanded towards the inclusion of chronic viral infections (including hepatitis B and C and HIV infections), and pioneering research on neurological disorders with suspected viral origin. Secondly, and in line with a more general trend in the life sciences, there has been a move from a focus on genomics towards the use of a broader spectrum of technologies and computation: 'a so-called integrative way of working [...] as given the complexity of the systems we study in biology, we need to combine existing and new technologies in our research' (interview with Andeweg, 2012). This also allows a shift towards virus discovery and identification, in addition to the understanding of viral infections and the development of anti-viral strategies. Similarly, the project organisation expanded from 14 to 19 partners: seven academic institutions, three research organisations and nine private sector companies. In parallel, also the management of the project expanded: 'While I started doing it alone, we now have a project management office of two to three people' (*idem*).

The prolongation of VIRGO I into VIRGO II shows the resilience of large-scale science projects as it proves difficult to break these new structures down again once they are in place (Lambright, 1998) but the end seems near as the project funds will finish in 2015: 'After that the dessert starts, then it is over. That is really true' (interview with Andeweg, 2012). The end seems final as the NGI dissolves completely in 2013, while VIRGO FES runs till 2015 – maybe allowing an extension till 2016 – but then also terminates as FES money will not be invested in research afterwards. This situation does not only provide VIRGO, but Dutch life sciences research in general with a dark funding future: 'We will have to see how things will develop [...] but it would be nice if it will not burn out like a candle, isn't it?' (*idem*).

Conclusion

The analysis of the VIRGO consortium shows the influence of the project format on research and its role in bringing different societal domains together. Next to the creation of common objectives and deliverables, the project connects the different 'modes of ordering' of academia, industry and government: specific agendas, structures, procedures, and timeframes that are fundamental to the stories

---

12   FES is the abbreviation of 'Fonds voor Economische Structuurversterking' which is a Dutch fund for the strengthening of the economical infrastructure which is sourced from the profit the Netherlands makes with its natural gas.

13   See also: http://www.genomics.nl/Research/GenomicsCentres/VIRGO.aspx and http://www.virgo.nl, retrieved 8 January 2012.

and actions of each specific domain (Law, 1994). The project accommodates the crossing of boundaries through the creation of a new structure, common procedures, and particular temporal and spatial orderings, thereby resolving tensions between the different modes of ordering, or at least finding a workable solution. As such, the project links various organisational structures, but also orchestrates different practices and procedures in the project proposal and later within the project management.

However, next to boundary crossing and the merging of different modes of ordering, the building of VIRGO also shows how boundaries become realigned or are kept steady. This can be seen for instance in the objectives of the project. Although the different parties involved have formulated a common goal, they maintain their own separate goals underneath the shared goal. In addition, the structure of the project still maintains boundaries between different domains; while the overall structure of VIRGO presents collaboration, the actual research takes place in separate Work Packages that only require specific researchers to work together so they can follow their own way of working. In addition, scientists have made procedures inside the project as simple as possible, trying to keep governmental bureaucracy outside of daily project activities. Finally, borders are protected on an individual level. While some individual scientists are able to cross boundaries between the different domains, others decide to stay put in the scientific domain or change to industry. As a result, projects have a different face on the level of management, the actual research practice, and the individual level of scientists: they enable the merge of science with governmental and industrial orderings, but the project structure also leaves room to protect the division between science and industry.

Nevertheless, the use of the project format in science also causes major tensions as the scientific order repeatedly becomes secondary to other ways of ordering. Most importantly, the project mode of working tries to make science a structured and controlled process, which opposes the unpredictable character of the research process. For example, the fact that research has to start with a clear-cut problem and concrete objective does not leave space for gradual scientific development or surprise which is characteristic for innovative scientific research. This tension is nicely illustrated by the obligation of scientists to predict the number of patents they expect to produce:

> We sometimes have a good laugh about these forms. If you can predict what will be the result of your research, you do not have to perform the research anymore [...] And they want it [the number of patents] specified per year. It is like having to predict in which city you will live 10 years from now and also knowing in which street and at which number [...] If I already knew, I would not be working in academia but I would work as an adviser to a company. (Interview with Andeweg, 2005)

Also with regard to other aspects such as output, time, and space, the scientific order has been compromised. For instance, the objectives of the VIRGO research shifted from academic publications to results that fit into the industrial mode of ordering aiming for patents. In addition, the project time followed the governmental mode of ordering as the evaluation of research complied with the annual political rhythm while ignoring the pace of scientific developments, and its termination is also caused by the governmental decisions to discontinue funding sources. Similarly, the national government space prevailed over the international scientific orientation. In such cases the intermingling of the three societal domains – science, industry, government – in the project format has more impact on scientific ordering than on the other orderings, a phenomenon called 'asymmetrical convergence' (Kleinman and Vallas, 2006).

When looking more precisely at practices of science and innovation it becomes clear that invention not only takes place with regard to development of new knowledge and applications but also importantly resides in organisational arrangements:

> inventiveness should not be equated with the development of novel artifacts, or indeed with novelty and innovation in general. Rather, inventiveness can be viewed as an index of the degree in which an object or practice is associated with opening up possibilities. In this view, scientific and technical objects and practices are inventive precisely in so far as they are aligned with inventive ways of thinking and doing and configuring and reconfiguring relations with other actors. (Barry, 2001: 211)

This begs the question if the project format allows enough inventiveness to harbour the possibilities of research. VIRGO is an 'innovative cluster', but does the implementation of the project format also result in an innovative arrangement of relations? In the analysis it became visible how VIRGO was inventive in opening up possibilities to get research funding and adapt the organisation of research to funding requirements and the projectification that comes with it. However, the project format also limited possibilities and relations from a scientific perspective, as the scientific order was repeatedly compromised. Perhaps the organisation of science should be more flexible than the current projectification allows, leaving room for inventive ways to configure and reconfigure relations and adapt the organisational form to specific research practices? The analysis of the VIRGO project has shown that when projectifying (health) science, it is important to realise the opportunities and limits it brings.

References

Adam, B. 2004. *Time*. Cambridge: Polity.

Barry, A. 2001. *Political Machines: Governing a Technological Society*. London: Athlone Press.

Berkhout, G. 2002. *Het Nederlands innovatiebeleid: Tijd voor vernieuwing?* Den Haag: Ministerie van Economische Zaken.

Bijker, W.E. 2006. The vulnerability of technological culture. In: Nowotny, H. (ed.) *Cultures of Technology and the Quest for Innovation.* New York: Bergahn Books, 52–69.

Boekholt, P., Meijer, I. and Vullings, W. 2001. *Evaluation of the Valorisation Activities of the Netherlands Genomics Initiative (NGI).* Amsterdam: Technopolis.

Borst, P. 2004. *Knot door bureaucratie.* NRC Handelsblad, April 3, 46.

Boston, J., Martin, J., Pallot, J. and Walsh, P. 1996. *Public Management: The New Zealand Model.* Oxford: Oxford University Press.

Brown, N., Rappert, B. and Webster, A. 2000. *Contested Futures: A Sociology of Prospective Techno-science.* Aldershot: Ashgate.

Cicmil, S. and Hodgson, D. 2006. *Making Projects Critical.* Basingstoke: Palgrave MacMillan.

Etzkowitz, H. and Leydesdorff, L. 2000. The dynamics of innovation: From national systems and "Mode 2" to a triple helix of university–industry–government relations. *Research Policy*, 29(2), 109–23.

Etzkowitz, H. and Webster, A. 1998. *Capitalizing Knowledge: New Intersections of Industry and Academia.* Albany, NY: State University of New York Press.

Etzkowitz, H. and Leydesdorff, L. 2003. Can 'the public' be considered as a fourth helix in university–industry–government relations? Report of the Fourth Triple Helix Conference. *Science and Public Policy*, 30(1), 55–61.

Ferlie, E., Ashburner, L., Fitzgerald, L. and Pettigrew, A. 1996. *New Public Management in Action.* Oxford: Oxford University Press.

Folstar, P. 2002. Editorial. *News@genomics.nl*, 1(3), 3.

Gieryn, T. 1983. Boundary-work and the demarcation of science from non-science: Strains and interests in the professional ideologies of scientists. *American Sociological Review*, 48, 781–95.

Gieryn, T. 1995. Boundaries of science. In: Jasanoff, S., et al. (eds) *Handbook of Science and Technology Studies.* Thousand Oaks: Sage, 293–443.

Gieryn, T.F. 1999. *Cultural Boundaries of Science: Credibility on the Line.* London: University of Chicago Press.

Guston, D.H. 2001. Special issue: Boundary organizations in environmental policy and science. *Science, Technology & Human Values*, 26(4), 399–531.

Hackett E.J., Amsterdamska, O., Lynch, M. and Wajcman, J. 2008. *The Handbook of Science and Technology Studies*, 3rd edition. Cambridge, MA: MIT Press.

Health Protection Agency 2006. *Influenza Pandemics of the 20th Century*, http://www.hpa.org.uk/infections/topics_az/influenca/pandemic/history.-htm, retrieved 29 October 2007.

Hessels, L., Horlings, E., Noyons, E. and Wouters, P. 2012. *Research Coordination by Intermediary Organizations.* Paper for EGOS Colloquium, 5–7 July in Helsinki.

Hessels, L. and Deuten, J. 2012. *Coördinatie van publiek-privaat onderzoek; Van variëteit naar maatwerk*. Den Haag: Rathenau Instituut.

Hodgson, D.E. 2004. Project work: The legacy of bureaucratic control in the post-bureaucratic organization. *Organization*, 11(1), 81–100.

Johnston, S., Skamene, E., Rima, B. and Melero, J. 2007. *External Research Review VIRGO Consortium 2006*, http://www.qanu.nl/comasy/uploadedfiles/-Virgo.pdf, retrieved 29 October 2007.

Kleinman, D.L. and Vallas, S. 2006. Contradiction in convergence: Universities and industry in the biotechnology field. In: Frickel, S. and Moore, K. (eds) *The New Political Sociology of Science: Institutions, Networks, and Power*. Madison, WI: The University of Wisconsin Press, 35–62.

Kolata, G. 1999. *Flu: The Story of the Great Influenza Pandemic of 1918 and the Search for the Virus That Caused It*. New York: Farrar, Straus and Giroux.

Lambright, H.W. 1998. Downsizing big science: Strategic choices. *Public Administration Review*, 58(3), 259–68.

Law, J. 1994. *Organizing Modernity*. Oxford: Blackwell.

van Lente, H. 1993. *Promising Technology: The Dynamics of Expectations in Technological Developments*. Enschede: Universiteit Twente.

Lock, D. 2003. *Project Management*, 8th edition. Aldershot: Gower Publishing.

Midler, C. 1995. Projectification of the firm: The renault case. *Scandinavian Journal of Management*, 11(4), 363–57.

NGI 2001. *The Netherlands Genomics Strategy. Strategic Plan 2002–2006*. The Hague: NGI.

NGI 2003. Dutch government awards Euro 86 million to NGI initiatives. *News@ genomics.nl*, 2(4), 11.

NGI 2005a. *Genomics 2008–2010: Bouwen en benutten; De Nederlandse genomics infrastructuur 2008–1012*. Den Haag: NGI.

NGI 2005b. *Netherlands Genomics Initiative, Annual Report 2004*. The Hague: NGI.

NGI 2005c. *Ondersteunende brieven*. Den Haag: NGI.

NGI 2005d. *Resultaten Nationale Genomics Strategie 2002–2007*. Den Haag: NGI.

NGI 2005e. VIRGO provides tools for anti-viral strategies. *News@genomics.nl*, 4(1), 4–5.

NGI 2006. *Strategic Plan Genomics 2008–2012*. The Hague: NGI.

NGI 2007a. *Businessplan NGI 2008–1012; Munt uit genomics*. Den Haag: NGI.

NGI 2007b. Dutch Cabinet awards NGI Euro 271 million. *Newsflash*, 18 September, http://www.genomics.nl/News%-20archive/18%20September%202007.aspx, retrieved 1 September 2008.

Parker, J.N., Vermeulen, N. and Penders, B. 2011. Admin burden is part of the job. *Nature*, 476(7358), 33.

Power, M. 1997. *The Audit Society: Rituals of Verification*. Oxford: Oxford University Press.

Quammen, D. 2012. Killers on the loose, the deadly viruses that threaten human survival. *The Guardian*, online 28 September, http://www.guardian. co.uk/society/2012/sep/28/deadly-viruses-ebola-marburg-sars, retrieved 30 September 2012.

de Rijck, K. 2005. Griepdreiging of bangmakerij. *De Standaard*, online 2 September, http://www.standaard.be/artikel/printartikel.aspx?artikelId-=GEFHGDUS, retrieved 1 December 2005.

Sahlin-Andersson, K. and Söderholm, A. 2002. *Beyond Project Management; New Perspectives on the Temporary–Permanent Dilemma*. Copenhagen: Liber.

Shapin, S. 2008. *The Scientific Life: A Moral History of a Late Modern Vocation*. Chicago, IL: The University of Chicago Press.

Shinn, T. 2002. The triple helix and new production of knowledge: Prepackaged thinking on science and technology. *Social Studies of Science*, 32(4), 599–614.

Shreeve, J. 2004. *The Genome War: How Craig Venter Tried to Capture the Code of Life and Save the World*. New York: Knopf.

Star, S. Leigh and Griesemer, J.R. 1989. Institutional ecology, 'translations' and boundary objects: Amateurs and professionals in Berkeley's Museum of Vertebrate Zoology. *Social Studies of Science*, 19(3), 387–421.

Torka, M. 2006. Die Projektförmigkeit der Forschung. *Die Hochschule*, 1, 63–83.

Venter, J.C. 2007. *A Life Decoded. My Genome: My Life*. New York: Viking.

Vermeulen, N. 2009. *Supersizing Science; On the Building of Large-scale Research Projects in Biology*. Maastricht: Maastricht University Press.

Weinberg, A.M. 1967. *Reflections on Big Science*. Oxford: Pergamon Press.

Whitley, R. 1984. *The Intellectual and Social Organization of the Sciences*. Oxford: Clarendon Press.

WHO 2005a. *Avian Influenza: Assessing the Pandemic Threat*, http://www.who. int/csr/-disease/influenza/H5N1–9reduit.pdf, retrieved 29 October 2007.

WHO 2005b. *WHO Global Influenza Preparedness Plan*. Geneva: WHO.

Chapter 4

Who Wants to Collaborate with Social Scientists? Biomedical and Clinical Scientists' Perceptions of Social Science

Mathieu Albert, Suzanne Laberge and Brian D. Hodges

Introduction

Interdisciplinarity and collaborative research seems to be the new creed of science policymakers, funding agencies, and university administrators in Canada. Many initiatives have been introduced to foster collaboration, both among academics and between academics and non-academic organizations (e.g., Government of Canada, 2001; Government of Alberta, 2005; Government of Manitoba, 2003; Government of Quebec, 2001). Major funding agencies have engaged in restructuring processes to break down the organizational boundaries between disciplines (e.g., Government of Canada, 2000; FQRSC, 2003; SSHRC, 2005) and several universities promote interdisciplinary research and training (e.g., McGill University, 2013; University of Toronto, 2012; University of Victoria, 2012; University of Western Ontario, 2001; York University 2005).

In health research, the growing interest of policymakers in interdisciplinarity has spawned initiatives to include the social sciences. For example, the Medical Research Council of Canada was replaced in 2000 by the Canadian Institutes for Health Research (CIHR) to promote collaborative research on a wide range of determinants of health, the name change signalling a broader range of methods and concerns than the traditional biological focus of 'medical' research. The new areas targeted by the CIHR include the cultural, social, economic, and environmental determinants of health (CIHR, 2003; 2005; Government of Canada, 2000). In a parallel development, clinical departments and research centres in Canadian medical schools have been hiring an increasing number of PhDs including social scientists (Fang and Meyer, 2003).

Although the idea of a greater role for the social sciences in health research looks promising, mandating change is not sufficient for effecting change. Studies, as well as accounts of social scientists doing research on health, suggest that current attempts to integrate the social sciences into the health research field are encountering difficulties (Béhague et al., 2008; Bernier, 2005; de Villier, 2005; Graham et al., 2011; Morse, 2005; 2006; Prainsack et al., 2010; Stokols, 2003). Difficulties arise in part because the social sciences must integrate into a domain in which experimental methods and randomized controlled trials are seen as 'gold standards' (Goldenberg, 2006; Holmes et al., 2006; Montgomery and Pool, 2011; Timmermans and Berg, 2003). Several medical anthropologists report that the predominance of the experimental and quasi-experimental paradigms creates a lack of parity between the social and the health sciences with regard to their perceived scientific authority (Barret, 1997; Foster, 1987; Kendall, 1989; Lambert and McKevitt, 2002; Napolitano and Jones, 2006). They stress that epidemiologists and clinical scientists perceive the social sciences as an activity of lower scientific value. As a result, social scientists tend to be confined to subordinate roles in interdisciplinary research teams and control relatively limited financial resources compared to clinical or biomedical investigators (see MacMynowski (2007) and Strang (2009) for similar report of power differential between the social sciences and the natural sciences in environmental research, and Parker (2010) for an analysis of the structural barriers hampering collaboration between ecologists and social scientists).

In light of these difficulties, certain pivotal questions need to be addressed: to what extent is it possible to create an interdisciplinary health research environment in which the social sciences can be fully integrated? Can the social sciences thrive in an environment in which the experimental paradigm occupies a hegemonic position and represents the epitome of science? To explore these questions, we investigated the perceptions and judgments of biomedical scientists and clinical scientists regarding the epistemology and methodologies characteristic of the social sciences.

Understanding the perceptions of biomedical and clinical scientists as they relate to the social sciences is critical because of the high status these groups typically hold in the health research field (at least in Canada), and consequently the symbolic power[1] they wield over it (Clarke, 2001; Clarke et al., 2003; Gordon, 1988). Although the goal of our study was not to empirically examine the enactment and impact of biomedical and clinical scientists' perceptions, we argue that those perceptions could function as boundary work (Gieryn, 1999), and affect social scientists' careers and integration in the health research field (e.g., their ability to access research funding, to network with other health scientists, to establish collaborative relationships and to achieve scientific legitimacy).

Our study of biomedical and clinical scientists' perceptions of social science research draws on Bourdieu's concepts of 'disciplinary habitus' (2004) and 'field' (1975; 1993; 2004). The concept of disciplinary habitus was developed to capture how scientific practices result from a socialization process. Disciplinary habitus involves the internalization, via disciplinary education and training, of schemes of perceptions, judgments and actions. This system of schemes provides cognitive categories for seeing/defining science, assessing 'good'/'bad' science, and carrying out scientific research in accordance with the standards in one's own discipline.

---

1 P. Bourdieu (1991) defines symbolic power as the power to make people see and believe certain visions of the world rather than others.

According to Bourdieu, the disciplinary habitus provides scientists with a practical sense of what has to be done and how it has to be done, so that they are perceived as legitimate scientists (Bourdieu, 2004). It includes knowing what research problems are important to investigate, what methodology will generate 'valid' results, what assessment criteria are appropriate, which journals are considered 'legitimate', and which conferences to attend. The practical sense varies according to the disciplinary education/socialization acquired. One of the ways a scientist's disciplinary habitus manifest itself is through his/her perception of, and position-taking on research practices in his/her own discipline as well as with regard to others. These perceptions may in turn work as a boundary by either including, excluding, ranking, etc., different scientific practices.

While acknowledging the heuristic usefulness of Bourdieu's concept of disciplinary habitus, it needs to be modified to suit the distinctiveness of the socialization process in the emerging interdisciplinary health research environment. Bourdieu's use of habitus aims to highlight the specific cultural schemes of scientific disciplines (e.g., chemistry and physics; Bourdieu, 2004: 37–44), and does not consider interdisciplinary research and training. Given that an increasing number of health scientists are being trained in an interdisciplinary research environment[2] or have moved from one discipline to another during their university training, we developed the concept of epistemic habitus to better grasp the non-disciplinary bounded health scientists' culture and practices. Our concept retains from Bourdieu the notion that scientists internalize cognitive categories through their academic training and professional experience. However, in contrast with Bourdieu's concept, epistemic habitus allows to move away from institutional disciplinary boundaries and focus on the broader common core of scientific trainings that transcends disciplinary borders. The experimental paradigm is part of the common core as it forms the main anchor for various types of health research training and practice, whether it be basic (biomedical) or applied (clinical). While the biomedical and clinical sciences differ significantly in the methods (see Knorr-Cetina (1999) on scientific cultures in basic sciences), both are grounded on the premise that the experimental method epitomizes legitimate research procedure.

To understand the power relations between groups of scientists with different habitus, we called upon Bourdieu's concept of 'field' (1975; 1993; 2004). A field refers to a hierarchical arena of social positions in which agents struggle for power (i.e. legitimacy and control over resources distribution). The health research domain can be seen as a field in which different groups of scientists interact, each of them wielding a certain degree of power. When newcomers enter a field – such as social scientists in the field of health – they can alter power relations in that field. Power relations play out around the key issues at stake in a given field. In the health

---

2   A growing number of health scientists are trained within, or are affiliated with, interdisciplinary programs or research centres (for example, public health, health promotion, system biology, proteomic, epigenetic, neuropsychiatry).

research field, the definition of 'legitimate' scientific research and the criteria for assessing research quality are key issues. Groups who succeed in imposing their criteria and research practices as legitimate hold authority in the field. Our study explores how two dominant groups, biomedical and clinical scientists, perceive the scientific practices of a third group, social scientists, entering the field of health research, and what boundaries these perceptions discursively create.

Methods

Sampling Procedure

To investigate biomedical and clinical scientists' perceptions and judgments of the social sciences we conducted semi-structured interviews with 61 biomedical scientists and clinical scientists who are members of peer review committees at the Canadian Institutes for Health Research (CIHR), which is a central Canadian health funding agency. We selected these scientists because members of peer review committees are generally considered by their peers to embody an institutionalized definition of scientific excellence (Guetzkow et al., 2004). Many are nominated by members of the broader research community to be panelists on these committees. Because those with scientific authority play a significant role in shaping the dominant vision of 'good science', their perception and judgment of social science is likely to be indicative of what is valued among biomedical and clinical scientists.

We used a sampling strategy that allowed us to maximize the diversity of perspectives from within each of the two academic communities of scientists and to explore the common and unique perspectives within and between the two groups (Sandelowski and Barosso, 2007). Accordingly, we targeted individuals from a range of research areas, peer-review committees, geographical locations, levels of seniority, and institutional affiliations (departments and universities). The number of respondents interviewed in each scientific community was determined by using a saturation approach: new participants were added to our sample until the variety of opinions was exhausted (Denzin and Lincoln, 2005). Our final sample consisted of 31 biomedical (i.e. laboratory) scientists and 30 clinical scientists. Table 4.1 summarizes the main characteristics of the sample.

The Interview Guide

We developed an interview guide with 34 semi-structured questions covering nine main themes. The following five themes were analyzed in greater detail for this chapter:

1. Exposure to the social sciences;
2. Research experience with social scientists;

Table 4.1   Main characteristics of the sample

	Biomedical Scientists n=31	Clinical Scientists n=30
Men	n=18	n=23
Women	n=13	n=7
Professor	n=17	n=17
Associate Professor	n=13	n=10
Assistant Professor	n=1	n=3
Number of Years as Faculty		
Median	14 years	20 years
Min–Max	4–31 years	1–34 years
Number of CIHR committees	n=20	n=15
Number of university affiliations	n=16	n=12

3. Opinions about different research methods: experimental, quasi-experimental, qualitative;
4. Opinions concerning the social sciences in the health domain;
5. Assessment of various types of methodology with respect to their bias and validity.

In addition, participants were asked to fill out a questionnaire on their socio-professional profile prior to the interview. Data from this questionnaire were considered in exploring the link between their perspectives on the social sciences and their training and academic trajectory as well as their exposure to the social sciences.

Data Collection

The interview script was sent to the participants prior to the interview. Most acquainted themselves with the questions before the interview. Interviews lasted between 60 and 90 minutes and were audio-recorded with the participants' consent. Phone interviews were used as the participants were affiliated with universities spread across Canada. Five pilot interviews were conducted before the study began to refine the interview guide.

Data Analysis

The data were analyzed by thematic content analysis. First, categories were generated reflecting the various positions expressed by all respondents with regard to each theme. Second, each interview was analyzed based on these categories (vertical analysis). Third, the data were examined from a comparative perspective across respondents (transversal analysis). Two investigators analyzed the interviews. Each one independently read and coded all interviews. Their respective coding structures were then compared. Any differences in interpretation were resolved through discussion until a consensus was obtained.

To get a synoptic overview of how receptive or unreceptive biomedical and clinical scientists were toward the social sciences, we converted into quantitative data some of the results of the qualitative analysis relating to respondents' perceptions of social science research. It must be stressed that the aim of this quantitative conversion was not to statistically test a hypothesis, but solely to provide an additional descriptive analysis that would help identify the major trends in biomedical and clinical scientists' receptiveness to the social sciences. Our quantification of the qualitative data proceeded as follows. First, a numerical value was attributed to the responses given by the participants to each of five semi-open questions targeting their perception of non-experimental methods (i.e., quantitative and qualitative social science methods) and the validity of the knowledge generated with these methods (see Appendix for the questions used). This was done using a five-point Likert-type scale with anchors that captured various degrees of receptiveness to the social sciences (1: unreceptive, 2: somewhat unreceptive, 3: ambivalent, 4: somewhat receptive, and 5: receptive). We assumed that biomedical and clinical scientists' perceptions and judgements of the methodologies characteristic of the social sciences would be a good entry point into their epistemic habitus. Moreover, given that biomedical and clinical scientists might not have been able to position themselves on either the substantive content or the theoretical relevance of social science research, methodological issues appeared to be the only common ground on which biomedical and clinical scientists could base their assessment of the scientific value of social science research. The construct sought in the use of the scale was that of positive or negative 'stance' toward the social sciences.

Because all respondents were asked to comment on issues related to non-experimental methods and the social sciences throughout the interview (i.e., except for the five selected questions that directly related to methods), we were also able to make an overall rating of how receptive the biomedical and clinical scientist participants were toward social science research. To do this, the same five-point scale was used to assign an overall score on the basis of the whole interview. By taking into account the entire context of the interview, we increased our confidence in the interpretation of the participants' responses to individual questions. Two investigators separately conducted the quantitative scoring. In the rare instances of discrepant scores, consensus was reached through discussion. We then proceeded to calculate, for each participant, the mean value of the six ratings in order to create a mean score reflecting his or her overall degree of receptiveness toward the social sciences. This mean score allowed us to position each respondent on a continuum ranging from 1 to 5, with 1 indicating a highly unreceptive posture or negative appraisal, and 5 a highly receptive posture or positive appraisal.

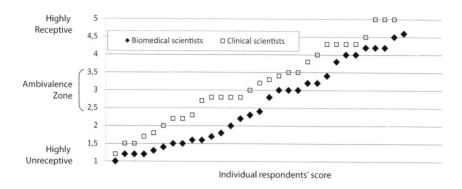

Figure 4.1 **Biomedical and clinical scientists' receptiveness score toward social science research**

Findings

First, we will present a portrait of biomedical and clinical scientists' general receptiveness to the social sciences. We will then focus on the rationale behind the biomedical and clinical scientists' level of receptiveness to the social sciences.

As Figure 4.1 shows, both clinical and biomedical scientists' receptiveness scores ranged widely, from a very negative stance to a very positive one. Neither group was homogeneous when it came to assessing social science research. However, clinical scientists tended to be somewhat more receptive to the social sciences than were biomedical scientists. While approximately half of the clinical scientists tended to be receptive to social science research, only one quarter of the biomedical scientists exhibited the same posture. Conversely, while approximately half of the biomedical scientists tended to be unreceptive toward the social sciences, only one quarter of the clinical scientists showed a similar unreceptiveness. We considered respondents with a score between 2.5 and 3.6 as ambivalent (see the Ambivalence Zone in Figure 4.1). Individuals within this range showed both favourable and unfavourable stances toward the social sciences depending on the specific issue addressed.

Biomedical and Clinical Scientists' Rationales for Receptiveness to Social Science Research

The content analysis revealed that biomedical and clinical scientists who were receptive to the social sciences used three arguments to support their posture. First, social science research questions are just as scientifically relevant as those of the biomedical and clinical sciences. Second, the methods typically used in the social sciences, both quantitative and qualitative, are as scientific and rigorous as those used in the biomedical and clinical sciences. Third, key aspects of health can only be studied by the social sciences. This last observation was often accompanied by an explicit recognition of the scientific legitimacy of the methods typically used in the social sciences:

> I think all methods have their place. And certainly the qualitative research addresses areas that are as important as those addressed by the basic sciences; they just do it with the methods that are appropriate in order to get at the answers. (07BMS)[3]

> In the clinical world we use randomized control trial, but many health issues cannot be answered by this and you need to use other approaches. (23CLS)

For most of the receptive biomedical and clinical scientists, the legitimacy of a method, whether it be experimental, quasi-experimental, quantitative or qualitative, essentially depends on its capacity to accurately address a research question, and not the degree to which it conforms to a given scientific paradigm. According to these scientists, there is no universal benchmark that would make it possible to determine the superiority of one method over another. Rather, as noted by several participants, the researcher must decide which method is the most appropriate for each particular question:

> The methods should be matched to the goals of your research. You need to ask yourself, what's most appropriate for getting the understanding that you need. Depending on the situation, non-experimental methods could be more appropriate. (03CLS)

> The method one uses is very much determined by the type of research one does. Researchers need to use the most appropriate method for the question they try to answer. Sometimes it may be an experimental approach sometimes it may be a qualitative approach as use in the social sciences. Establishing a hierarchy of methods is probably a narrow view on how to do research. (13BMS)

> There are some types of questions that just aren't amenable to experimental approaches, and not just because they're in the early stages. Because they would never be anything other than something you have to get qualitative answers to. (06BMS)

Many of the receptive biomedical and clinical scientists showed a critical posture toward their own research practices, whether they engage in laboratory sciences or clinical research, such as randomized controlled trials (RCTs) and clinical

---

3   The code in parenthesis following each interview quote corresponds to the respondent's identification number.

epidemiology. This self-reflective attitude may support openness to other types of scientific practices, such as those of the social sciences. Receptive participants acknowledged that there is an element of subjectivity and interpretation in both the experimental/clinical sciences and the social sciences. In their view, subjectivity and interpretation are to be found in the experimental and clinical sciences in three main areas: (1) the framework used to inform the research question and interpret the results, (2) the technical apparatus and data collection procedures, and (3) the scientist's subjective decision regarding what is appropriate to do at the various steps of the research. The following quotes illustrate participants' perspectives:

> I don't buy into the argument that because something is numeric it's objective. I mean, it's only as objective as the way you appraise, the way you design the numeric question. (06BMS)

> I think there is good science and bad science. Almost all science has some bias. There is no perfect science. I think there are lousy biomedical scientists and there are lousy social scientists. The best social science is probably pretty good stuff. Maybe I'm wrong, but I don't see a big difference between experimental and social sciences. I don't think they should be treated differently. (10CLS)

> Medical scientists are sort of very full of themselves, and they think that what they are doing is the best without looking into the other things. I don't think that's right. (05CLS)

Interestingly, many receptive biomedical and clinical scientists acknowledged that their studies do not measure reality as it is and do not provide an unmediated account of it. They acknowledged that the 'controlled' environments they create are artificial and the conclusions they generate are actually interpretations based on hypotheses and on the state of knowledge at the time of carrying out the research. In this sense these respondents leaned toward a constructivist/rationalist epistemology more than to a positivist or empiricist one (Bachelard, 1980; Bourdieu et al., 1991). The following two quotes illustrate the majority opinion among the receptive biomedical and clinical scientists about the constructed nature of scientific results:

> How you choose to ask a question, what you choose to report, how you choose to present it inherently changes the results in the way we view it. Data don't speak by themselves because how we interpret them depends on the references upon which we interpret them. (25BMS)

> Everything is a construction, there's no such thing as truth. There's only truth in religion. Everything's is a construction consistent with a hypothesis. So, truth is for believers, it's not for scientists. (10BMS)

With regard to collaboration with social scientists, one may argue that the receptive biomedical and clinical scientists would likely be open to such prospect. Indeed, as we will see further in the paper, some of them have collaborated or were collaborating with social scientists at the time of the interview. These collaborations may have fostered their receptiveness to research methodologies different from their own and incline them to be inclusive of social science research.

Biomedical and Clinical Scientists' Rationales for Unreceptiveness to Social Science Research

Biomedical and clinical scientists who showed a low level of receptiveness to the social sciences (17 out of the 31 biomedical scientists, and 7 out of the 30 clinical scientists; see Figure 4.1) anchored their stance in a strict definition of 'legitimate' science. This definition was characterized by three key assumptions: (1) the best science necessarily involves the performance of an intervention on variables; (2) this intervention must be done in a controlled environment[4] or with a randomized sample[5] to permit the establishment of a causal or correlational relationship; (3) results must be reproducible to ensure that they are not due to chance. Given that the social sciences, and more particularly qualitative research, cannot satisfy these criteria, the unreceptive respondents hold them to be unscientific.

Consistent with their definition of legitimate science, unreceptive biomedical and clinical scientists asserted that there is a hierarchy among research methods. In their opinion, the experimental method is at the top of the hierarchy because it epitomizes legitimate scientific procedures. Results from experimental research are both valid and objective because they are produced in a controlled or quasi-controlled environment and are observable by any scientist performing the same experiment. Quantitative social research and epidemiology were ranked second – primarily by biomedical scientists (who rarely or never use them), and to a lesser degree by clinical scientists (who use them regularly). Although quantitative social research and epidemiology build on reliable methods and generate quantified and objective results, their statistical analyses only allow the establishment of correlations among variables rather than causal relationships. This was perceived as a weakness – mostly by biomedical scientists – since the goal of science, according to these scientists, is to uncover the causes of the observed phenomena. Qualitative research is ranked last by both the unreceptive biomedical and clinical scientists. They perceived it as being devoid of any scientific foundation for three main reasons: it cannot be reproduced; the researcher's subjectivity interferes at all stages of the research process which critically decrease their validity; and

---

4   A position predominantly held by biomedical scientists.
5   A position predominantly held by clinical scientists.

there is no effective way to control for bias. The following quotes are typical of unreceptive scientists' rationale for their ranking:

> There are objective methods for assessing the validity of experimental data, and objective methods for analyzing quantitative data where there are fewer methods to do things like that in qualitative research. And also, by definition, qualitative research is very much influenced by the set-up of the information gathering: by the way you set up your interview and the way the questions are read, or the way the questions are posed. That has huge effects on the outcome. These are very difficult to control. Whereas in experimental and quantitative methods, you can go back and change a parameter if you realize that something was not controlled. You cannot go back and give the same interview again, changing the questions, because having heard the questions before, the subject is already changed. (09BMS)

> There is more risk of error in qualitative research and the social sciences than there is in quantitative methods because the precision tends to be softer. It would be bad for anyone to do a qualitative research without any quantification because the end results would merely be opinions which may or may not be correct. I look at qualitative studies as hypothesis generating. If it is used that way then I have no problem. But if you use qualitative research and you claim that you are going to generate data to support your hypothesis, I think you are going to get into trouble. (28CLS)

> I don't know very much about social sciences and that kind of research. But part of the reason why I think there is a hierarchy is because I like things to be objective and quantitative as much as possible. People who do quantitative research kind of control things very well. Sometimes it seems that with non-quantitative research you can almost get the result you want. (26BMS)

In contrast to their colleagues who grant legitimacy to the social sciences, the unreceptive biomedical and clinical scientists did not endorse the idea that one may use different methods depending on the nature of the research question. For them, research questions that do not lend themselves to laboratory experimentation (a position predominantly held by biomedical scientists) or experimental analysis such as in RCT or epidemiological study (a position predominantly held by clinical scientists) cannot be studied in a scientific manner.

Based on the view expressed by the unreceptive scientists, it is likely that collaboration with social scientists would be difficult to establish. Indeed, it would be challenging for these scientists to engage in collaborative work with individuals who use research methods they don't consider scientific. The epistemic habitus they internalized during their academic training and career path seems to incline them to draw a boundary between what they define as legitimate science (their own research practice) and what is not (the social scientists' research practice).

Biomedical and Clinical Scientists' Rationales for an Ambivalent Posture toward Social Science Research

Like the unreceptive respondents, ambivalent biomedical and clinical scientists tended to exhibit a hierarchical view of science: they placed the experimental method at the top of the hierarchy and qualitative research at the bottom because they perceived experimental method to be more reliable and to generate more valid result than qualitative methods. For many of the ambivalent respondents the methodological limitation of qualitative methods constitutes a sensitive issue affecting their receptiveness to the social sciences. However, in contrast to the unreceptive respondents, these participants viewed all forms of inquiry, including qualitative research, as scientific endeavours. In their view, there is no cut-off point at which academic research practice falls outside the scientific field. The boundary they establish manifests itself through the ranking of the different research practices in the field rather than through the exclusion of the non-experimental research practices. The following quotes exemplify their hierarchized view of scientific practice:

> There's probably more potential for bias in the qualitative research because the investigator is putting more of himself into the process of questionnaires so it's a more subjective interpretation. It doesn't mean it's necessarily bad, it just means that you have to be a bit careful about avoiding and recognizing what potential biases there could be. (30CLS)

> Where the method is amenable to statistics you can be a lot less arbitrary in what you say, but if there is no other way of doing the research than using qualitative methods one has to be happy with it. (13BMS)

> I respect qualitative methods but there are issues of generalizability which I feel are very important which I don't think they approach very well. (22CLS)

In terms of collaboration with social scientists, it is likely that the ambivalent biomedical and clinical scientists would engage in such work, but potentially on the condition that quantitative methods are preferred over qualitative ones.

Link between Exposure and Receptivity to the Social Sciences

How can we understand the variation in the biomedical and clinical scientists' receptiveness toward the social sciences? To shed light on the variation we explored the respondents' professional trajectory focusing on their exposure to the social sciences. In line with our concept of epistemic habitus (the claims that scientists' views on science result from their academic socialization and career experience), our assumption was that biomedical and clinical scientists who had

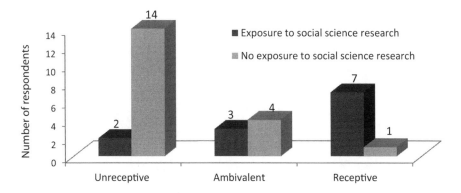

Figure 4.2   Biomedical scientists' receptivity to social science according to their exposure to social science research

been exposed to social science research (for example by working collaboratively with social scientists, participating in the development of social science research projects, or evaluating such kind of project as a member of an interdisciplinary peer review committee) would show a greater receptiveness to the social sciences than those who had not. To get an overview of the possible link between exposure and receptiveness to social sciences research, we graphically represented the connection between these two themes, separately for biomedical and clinical scientists. Our goal here is solely to highlight the potential link between exposure and receptiveness yielded by the interview data and participants' training and career trajectory (to which we had access through their CV), not to test an hypothesis.

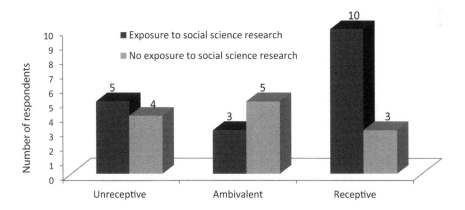

Figure 4.3   Clinical scientists' receptivity to social science according to their exposure to social science research

For both groups of scientists (see Figure 4.2 and Figure 4.3), results suggest that most of the receptive respondents have been exposed to social science (7 of the 8 receptive biomedical scientists and 10 of the 13 receptive clinical scientists).

Participants' comments explicitly attributed their own receptiveness to their prior experiences engaging with social scientists as collaborators on interdisciplinary research projects or as panellists on interdisciplinary peer review committees. As the following accounts suggest, these experiences seem to have generated favourable perceptions of the social sciences:

> I started to look differently at the social sciences when I participated on an interdisciplinary peer-reviewed committee and when I started collaborating with a social scientist. I realized the importance of the work done in this area and started to appreciate the interesting point of view social scientists brought to research. (24BMS)

> I have developed a very positive view on social scientists. I was naïve going in and my colleague who is a social scientist did a lot to open my eyes. I was trained as a quantitative clinician-scientist and he taught me lots about qualitative research. I now see the complementarities of qualitative and quantitative research. I think I've been educated. (05CLS)

Conversely, our data suggest, that only few unreceptive respondents have been exposed to social sciences, notably among the biomedical scientists (2 of 16). The interviews suggest that their university education played a key role in shaping their scientific belief and epistemic habitus:

> My Bachelor is in Chemistry, my Master's in Biochemistry and my PhD in Molecular Biology. I've been taught during all my university training that there is a hierarchy in research methods and that the experimental method is best. That's the way I see things now. (20BMS)

> I have been trained in basic sciences. Therefore, I have been taught a method of science that demands experimental testing of hypotheses. Therefore I mainly believe in the scientific rigor of the experimental method. (25BMS).

> I [learned] through my training that the scientific method requires that you can reproduce it, that another person can come along, use the same methodology and come up with the same results. If it's qualitative, that's not going to happen because there is the qualitative component. That's an issue. (17CLS)

The link between exposure and receptiveness to social science seems to be less obvious in the clinical scientists (see Figure 4.3). The results indicate a similar number of unreceptive respondents who have been exposed (n=5) and not exposed (n=4) to social science. While we were careful to ascertain saturation of emergent themes, including around the issue of exposure/stance, it is possible that further interviewing might uncover additional factors related to receptiveness. Despite this caveat, interview data nevertheless suggest that the 'quality' of the interaction may be playing a role in scientists' receptiveness. Some clinical scientists reported that they had an unconstructive experience when interacting with social scientists and that has affected their receptiveness. The following quote from a clinical scientist illustrates such experience:

> My collaboration with social scientists showed me that we really do not share the same scientific language. Their theoretical jargon is confusing and counterproductive. I would be reluctant to engage again into collaborative work with a social scientist. (30CLS)

Therefore, it is likely that simply being exposed may not be sufficient to develop receptiveness to social science. The quality of the collaboration experience may be a significant feature that also needs to be taken into account to understand the link between exposure and receptiveness to social science.

Discussion and Conclusion

In the current move toward interdisciplinary health research, it is critical to understand how scientists from different backgrounds perceive and judge one another. Perceptions can shape attitudes toward collaborative work, and direct resources toward specific types of research practices and methodologies and not to others. The majority of the studies and essays exploring the relationship between social and medical scientists have focused on social scientists' difficulties functioning within interdisciplinary research teams (Béhague et al., 2008; Bernier, 2005; de Villier, 2005; Barret, 1997; Foster, 1987; Lambert and McKevitt, 2002; Napolitano and Jones, 2006). Although it is important to have an appreciation of the challenges faced by social scientists on interdisciplinary teams, we contend that it is also critical to explore the perceptions and judgments of the dominant scientific groups (the biomedical and clinical scientists) given that their perceptions and judgments may act as a symbolic boundary (Albert et al., 2009; Gieryn, 1999). This study explored the biomedical and clinical scientists' perceptions of the scientific value of social sciences.

Our study has shown that many biomedical and clinical scientists hold predominantly an unfavourable or ambivalent posture toward social science research. However, our findings also indicate that neither group of scientists is homogeneous with regard to their perspective on social science research. First, both clinical and biomedical scientists' receptiveness scores ranged widely, from a very negative to a very positive posture. Second, we observed that clinical scientists tended to be more receptive to the social sciences than their biomedical colleagues.

Moreover, results of our analyses suggest that exposure to social science research is a salient theme in biomedical and clinical scientists' rationales regarding receptiveness to the social sciences. In our view, this brings some support to our hypothesis according to which scientific training and professional experience (including exposure to other scientific paradigms) may shape one's perception and judgements toward scientific practices. While the biomedical and clinical scientists may have acquired an experimental epistemic habitus during their university education, the majority who had been exposed to social science research may have had their habitus altered in the sense of an enlarging of their perspective on scientific practices and an acknowledging of the legitimacy of the social sciences. Those results are consistent with recent studies showing that biomedical scientists' perceptions of social sciences changed after working with social scientists (Jeffrey, 2003; Stokols et al., 2003). However, our findings also highlighted that exposure may not be sufficient to develop receptiveness to social science; the quality of the collaboration experience seems to be an important feature that also needs to be taken into account to understand the link between exposure and receptiveness to social science. Further research is needed to better grasp the impact of the positive or negative collaboration experience on clinical and biomedical receptiveness to social science.

The reservations expressed by the ambivalent biomedical and clinical scientists about qualitative methods suggest that the perspective on science they initially internalized remains well-grounded and continues to function as the generating principle of their perceptions and judgments. In her study on interdisciplinary scholarship, Lattuca (2001) also observed the enduring influence of disciplinary training on the ways researchers approach a research problem. She pointed out that even those who had a long engagement with interdisciplinary scholarship tend to fall back into their 'disciplinary habit of mind' (2001: 225).

Looking at the data through the lens of Bourdieu's concept of field (1975; 2004), social scientists can be viewed as newcomers entering into a field structured by power relations where the biomedical and clinical scientists and their scientific culture hold a hegemonic position. Social scientists' research practices will be judged according to the epistemic categories of the dominant groups. Thus their value is likely to be determined by those who hold the power to define what is or is not valuable in the field. Dominant scientific standards may thus act as a boundary work.

In conclusion, our findings suggest that social scientists have limited support from health research scientists. This limited support may be an impediment for social scientists to engage in collaborative research work with biomedical and clinical scientists, and gain status in the health research field. This provides further evidence for the claim made by medical anthropologists (Barret, 1997; Foster, 1987; Lambert and McKevitt, 2002; Napolitano and Jones, 2006) that social scientists working in health tend to be confined to subordinate roles. Our findings also resonate with those of MacMynowski (2007) and Strang (2009) who reported power imbalance between social science and natural science in environmental research.

In order to better grasp the social dynamic of knowledge production in the broad health research field, future research should investigate the definition of legitimate science advocated by other scientific communities, such as epidemiologists, health services researchers, and medical humanities scholars, and their power relationships with one another. These definitions and these power relationships are likely to shape the field and create either fertile or unfertile conditions for collaboration. Moreover, building on our results, future research should aim at better measuring the extent to which exposure to social science research (or to any other types of scientific inquiry) and the quality of the experience lead to a greater receptiveness, and which may, in turn, induce a favourable attitude toward interdisciplinary collaboration.

Acknowledgement

This research was supported by the Canadian Institutes of Health Research, grant # KTE-72140. We wish to thank the participants for giving their time to this study.

Appendix

Questions used to construct the receptiveness score:

- 'Many health researchers believe that there is a hierarchy of research methods, which is determined by the methodology's rigor. Do you agree that there is this hierarchy? Explain'.
- 'Some researchers think that qualitative research (such as studies using interviews or focus groups) is mainly to be used in the preliminary phases of quantitative research. Do you agree that this should be the primary use of qualitative methods? Explain'.
- 'Do you think that there are more sources of bias within the social sciences than in the experimental sciences or is it equal? Explain'.
- 'Do you think the fact that the social sciences (or qualitative research) are subject to a greater number of bias compromises the validity of their results? Explain'.
- 'The *British Medical Journal* has proposed a checklist to assess the scientific value of qualitative studies in the health sciences (Mays and Pope, 1995). In the box below, five of these criteria are listed. Please give me your opinion on each of them. Do you think these are appropriate criteria for assessing qualitative research?' Our analysis has only scored the following 5th criterion: 'Did the investigator make use of quantitative evidence to test qualitative conclusions where appropriate? Explain'.

References

Albert, M., Laberge, S. and Hodges, B.D. 2009. Boundary work in the health research field: Biomedical and clinician scientists' perceptions of social science research. *Minerva*, 47(2), 171–94.

Bachelard, G. 1980. *La formation de l'esprit scientifique*. Paris: Vrin.

Barrett, B. 1997. Identity, ideology and inequality: Methodologies in medical anthropology, Guatemala 1950–1995. *Social Science & Medicine*, 44(5), 579–87.

Béhague, D., Pareja, G.H. and Gomes, V.C. 2008. Anthropology and epidemiology: Learning epistemological lessons through a collaborative venture. *Ciênca & Saúde Coletiva*, 13(6), 1701–10.

Bernier, N.F. 2005. Integrating political science into health sciences. In: Canadian Institutes of Health Research (ed.) *The Social Sciences and Humanities in Health Research*. Ottawa, 124–5.

Bourdieu, P. [2001] 2004. *Science of Science and Reflexivity*, Richard Nice (trans.). Cambridge, UK: Polity Press.

Bourdieu, P. 1993. *Sociology in Question*. London: Sage.

Bourdieu, P. 1991. *Language and Symbolic Power*. Cambridge, UK: Cambridge University Press.

Bourdieu, P. 1975. The specificity of the scientific field and the social conditions of the progress of reason. *Social Science Information*, 14(6), 19–47.

Bourdieu, P., Chamboredon, J.-C. and Passeron, J.-C. [1973] 1991. *The Craft of Sociology: Epistemological Preliminaries*. Berlin, New York: Walter de Gruyter.

CIHR 2005. *The Social Sciences and Humanities in Health Research* [Canadian Institutes of Health Research], http://publications.gc.ca/collections/collection_2007/cihr-irsc/MR21–58–2005E.pdf, retrieved 14 June 2013.

CIHR 2003. *Investing in Canada's Future: CIHR's Blueprint for Health Research and Innovation* [Canadian Institutes of Health Research], http://publications.gc.ca/collections/Collection/MR21–47–2004E.pdf, retrieved 14 June 2013.

Clarke, A. 2001. *The Sociology of Health Care*. New York: Prentice.

Clarke, A.E., Shim, J.K., Mamo, L., Fosket, J.R. and Fishman, J.R. 2003. Biomedicalization: Technoscientific transformations of health, illness, and US biomedicine. *American Sociological Review*, 68(2), 161–94.

Denzin, N.K. and Lincoln, Y.S. 2005. *The Sage Handbook of Qualitative Research*. Thousand Oaks: Sage.

De Villiers, J. 2005. Integrating the techniques of linguistic discourse into health sciences. In: Canadian Institutes of Health Research (ed.) *The Social Sciences and Humanities in Health Research*. Ottawa, 122–3.

Fang, D. and Meyer, R.E. 2003. PhD faculty in clinical departments of U.S. medical schools, 1981–1999: Their widening presence and role in research. *Academic Medicine*, 78(2), 167–76.

Foster, G.M. 1987. World Health Organization behavioral science research: Problems and prospects. *Social Science & Medicine*, 24(9), 709–17.

FQRSC–Fonds québécois de la recherche sur la société et la culture 2003. *Orientations stratégiques 2002–2005*. Québec City. http://www.frqsc.gouv. qc.ca/upload/publications-fqrsc/fichiers/publication_32.pdf, retrieved 14 June 2013.

Gieryn, T.F. 1999. *Cultural Boundaries of Science. Credibility on the Line*. Chicago: The University of Chicago Press.

Goldenberg, M.J. 2006. On evidence-based medicine: Lessons from the philosophy of science. *Social Science & Medicine*, 62(11), 2621–32.

Gordon, D.R. 1988. Clinical science and clinical expertise: Changing boundaries between art and science in medicine. In: M. Lock and D.R. Gordon (eds) *Biomedicine Examined*. Dordrecht: Kluwer, 257–95.

Government of Alberta 2005. *Innovation and Science. Business Plan, 2005–08*. Edmonton. http://www.finance.alberta.ca/publications/Budget/budget2005/innov.pdf, retrieved 14 June 2013.

Government of Canada 2001. *Achieving Excellence. Investing in people, Knowledge and Opportunity. Canada's Innovation Strategy*. Ottawa. http://publications. gc.ca/collections/Collection/C2-596-2001E.pdf, retrieved 14 June 2013.

Government of Canada 2000. *Bill C-13. An Act to Establish the Canadian Institutes of Health Research*. Ottawa. http://publications.gc.ca/pub?id=91491&sl=0, retrieved 14 June 2013.

Government of Manitoba 2003. *Manitoba at the Forefront of Innovation*. Winnipeg.

Government of Quebec 2001. *Knowledge to Change the World*. Québec City.

Graham, J., Adelson, N., Fortin, S., Bibeau, G., Lock, M., Hyde, S., Macdonald, M.H., Olazabal, I., Stephenson, P. and Waldram, J. 2011. A manifesto. The end of medical anthropology in Canada? *University Affairs*, March 2011, 37.

Guetzkow, J., Lamont, M. and Mallard, G. 2004. What is originality in the humanities and the social sciences? *American Sociological Review*, 69(2), 190–212.

Holmes, D., Stuart, J., Perron, A. and Rail, G. 2006. Deconstructing the evidence-based discourse in health sciences: Truth, power and fascism. *International Journal of Evidence-Based Health Care*, 4(3), 180–86.

Jeffrey, P. 2003. Smoothing the waters: Observations on the process of cross-disciplinary research collaboration. *Social Studies of Science*, 33(4), 539–62.

Kendall, C. 1989. The use and non-use of anthropology: The diarrheal disease control program in Honduras. In: J.V. Willigen, B. RylkoBauer and A. McElroy (eds) *Making Our Research Useful*. Boulder, CO: Westview, 283–303.

Knorr-Cetina, K. 1999. *Epistemic Cultures. How the Sciences Make Knowledge*. Cambridge, MA: Harvard University Press.

Lambert, H. and McKevitt, C. 2002. Anthropology in health research: From qualitative methods to multidisciplinary. *British Medical Journal*, 325, 210–13.

Lattuca, L.R. 2001. *Creating Interdisciplinarity*. Nashville: Vanderbilt University Press.

MacMynowski, D.P. 2007. Pausing at the brink of interdisciplinarity: Power and knowledge at the meeting of social and biophysical science. *Ecology and Society*, 12(1), 1–14.

Mays, N. and Pope, C. 1995. Qualitative research: Rigour and qualitative research. *British Medical Journal*, 311, 109–12.

McGill University 2013. *Strategic Research Plan* [Office of the Vice-Principal], http://www.mcgill.ca/research/sites/mcgill.ca.research/files/srp_long_ version_final_1.pdf, retrieved 14 June 2013.

Montgomery, C.M. and Pool, R. 2011. Critically engaging: Integrating the social and the biomedical in international microbicides research. *Journal of the International AIDS Society*, 14(Suppl. 2): S4, http://www.ncbi.nlm.nih.gov/ pmc/articles/PMC3194163/, retrieved 14 June 2013.

Morse, J.M. 2005. Beyond the clinical trial: Expanding criteria for evidence. *Qualitative Health Research*, 15(1), 3–4.

Morse, J.M. 2006. It is time to revise the Cochrane criteria. *Qualitative Health Research*, 16(3), 315–17.

Napolitano, D.A., and Jones, C.O.H. 2006. Who needs 'pukka' anthropologists? A study of the perceptions of the use of anthropology in tropical public health research. *Tropical Medicine and International Health*, 11(8), 1264–75.

Parker, J.N. 2010. Integrating the social into the ecological: Organizational and research group challenges. In: J.N. Parker, N. Vermulen and B. Penders (eds) *Collaboration in the New Life Sciences*. Farnham, UK: Ashgate, 85–109.

Prainsack, B., Svendsen, M.N., Koch, L. and Ehrich, K. 2010. How do we collaborate? Social science researchers' experience of multidisciplinarity in biomedical settings. *BioSocieties*, 5(2), 278–86.

Sandelowski, M. and Barroso, J. 2007. *Handbook for Synthesizing Qualitative Research*. Springer: New York.

SSHRC 2005. *Strategic Plan 2006–2011* [Social Sciences and Humanities Research Council of Canada], http://www.sshrc-crsh.gc.ca/about-au_sujet/ publications/framing_our_direction_e.pdf, retrieved 14 June 2013.

Stokols, D., Fuqua, J., Gress, J., Harvey, R., Phillips, K., Baezconde-Garbanati, L., Unger, J., Palmer, P., Clark, M.A., Colby, S.M., Morgan, G., and Trochin, W. 2003. Evaluating transdisciplinary science. *Nicotine & Tobacco Research*, 5, S21-S39.

Strang, V. 2009. Integrating the social and the natural sciences in environmental research: A discussion paper. *Environment and Sustainable Development*, 11(1), 1–18.

Timmermans, S. and Berg, M. 2003. *The Gold Standard: The Challenge of Evidence-Based Medicine and Standardization in Health Care*. Philadelphia: Temple University Press.

University of Toronto 2012. *Excellence, Leadership, Innovation. University of Toronto Research Strategic Plan 2012–1017*, http://www.research.utoronto. ca/strategic-initiatives/strategic-research-plan/, retrieved 14 June 2013.

University of Victoria 2012. *A Vision for the Future – Building on Excellence A Strategic Plan for the University of Victoria*, http://web.uvic.ca/strategicplan/pdf/strategic.pdf, retrieved 14 June 2013.

University of Western Ontario 2001. *Making Choices: Western's Commitments as a Research-Intensive University. Report of the Strategic Planning Task Force*, http://www.uwo.ca/univsec/SPTF2001/, retrieved 14 June 2013.

York University 2005. *University Academic Plan. Academic Priorities 2005–2010. The Senate of York University*, http://www.yorku.ca/secretariat/documents/UAP%202005–2010%20For%20Web.pdf, retrieved 14 June 2013.

Chapter 5

Credible to Collaborators Themselves: How Corporations and Trade Associations Made Trans Fats into a Problem

David Schleifer

When corporations and trade associations work together to conduct research specifically designed to protect their economic interests, who could believe their findings? Based on a discussion of two pivotal pieces of research about trans fats, I show that industry collaborators themselves are likely to believe the findings that they work together to produce. Furthermore, corporations and trade associations can decide to change their business strategies and technologies as a result of the findings they collaborate in producing. In other words, collaboration can result in the production of scientific claims that are credible to collaborators themselves and that can serve as the basis for changing industry actors' economic interests.[1]

Trans fats are a type of dietary fat created by processing liquid oil, usually soybean oil, using a method called partial hydrogenation.[2] In 2006, the United States Food and Drug Administration (FDA) mandated that manufacturers list trans fat content on the nutrition labels of packaged foods (FDA, 2003). The agency developed this labeling rule in response to a 1994 petition by a health advocacy organization called the Center for Science in the Public Interest (CSPI, 1994). Also in 2006, New York City banned trans fats from all restaurants and food service operations (Angell et al., 2009). Several other US cities followed suit (DeSoucey and Schleifer, 2010). In 2013, the FDA proposed new regulations that would effectively ban partially hydrogenated oils, citing 2005 a conclusion by the Institute of Medicine at the National Academies of Science that trans fats raise risk factors for heart disease (FDA, 2013b; IOM/NAS, 2005). The FDA's 2013 proposed ban noted that many food manufacturers had voluntarily replaced partially hydrogenated oils in their products since labeling took effect in 2006 and that trans fat consumption had fallen substantially (FDA, 2013a; Doell et al., 2012). Nonetheless, the FDA proposed that partially hydrogenated oils should be eliminated entirely from the US food system.

---

1   This chapter draws from research based on interviews with academic and industry scientists, nutritionists, health advocates and other professionals; as well as content analysis of scientific articles, policy documents and media reports.

2   Scientists typically italicize the trans in trans fats. To reduce visual distraction, I italicize it only when quoting texts that do so.

But views on partially hydrogenated oils and the trans fats they contain were very different 30 years ago. Throughout the 1980s, CSPI and another organization, the National Heart Savers Association (NHSA) pressured food manufacturers to remove saturated fats from their products based on the argument that saturated fats increase risk factors for heart diseases by raising "bad" LDL cholesterol. CSPI endorsed trans fats as a healthy or at least benign replacement for saturated fat (detailed in Schleifer, 2012). For example, in 1986 McDonalds replaced the saturated fats in some of its products with partially hydrogenated oils, the major source of trans fats. CSPI described this change as "a great gift to consumers' arteries" and "a responsible reaction to public pressure" (Jacobson and Fritschner, 1986). CSPI based its position on an apparent scientific consensus about the harmlessness of trans fats. The National Research Council at the National Academies of Science concluded in 1989 that trans fats had no effect on cholesterol (National Research Council, 1989). And a 1990 Institute of Medicine report determined that trans fats had "no deleterious effects" on human health (Institute of Medicine, 1990).

Yet by 2013, a team of Dutch academic scientists could confidently write that "the detrimental effects of industrial trans fatty acids on heart health are beyond dispute" (Brouwer et al., 2013). Two pieces of collaborative research, published in 1990 and 1994, precipitated this comprehensive reversal of views on trans fats. In the first piece of research, Martijn Katan, one of the aforementioned Dutch scientists, and his graduate assistant Ronald Mensink studied the effects on trans fats on humans. They did so in collaboration with Unilever, which provided them with margarines that they fed to their research subjects. Mensink and Katan concluded that trans fats raised risk factors for heart disease more than saturated fats did by both increasing LDL cholesterol and lowering "good" HDL cholesterol (Mensink and Katan, 1990).

Mensink and Katan's findings were published in the *New England Journal of Medicine* in 1990. Representatives of the US food, edible oil and soybean industries argued that the Dutch team's findings were misleading because the amount of trans fats in Dutch margarine was higher than in American margarines and because the method of producing them was different from that typically used in the United States. Therefore, a group of US trade associations and corporations collaborated on a second piece of research. They funded and provided materials to Joseph Judd and his team of researchers at a United States Department of Agriculture (USDA) laboratory, hoping that he would prove trans fats were safe. But Judd and his colleagues also found that trans fats raised LDL and lowered HDL cholesterol (Judd et al., 1994). CSPI, citing an advance copy of Judd et al.'s industry-funded research, petitioned the FDA for trans fat labeling in 1994. Industry actors began work on trans fat alternatives. The move against trans fats had begun.

Compromised Science?

These collaborations by academic and government researchers with corporations and trade associations may seem like prototypical examples of what Vallas and

Kleinman describe as the troubling blurring of boundaries between corporate and academic research (Vallas and Kleinman, 2007). This blurring of boundaries has a specific history. US government policies in the late 1970s began to recast academic science as potentially economically valuable, resulting in a range of new collaborative practices between academic and industrial institutions, including more research partnerships between corporations and universities (Berman, 2012). Financial conflicts of interest can have troubling effects on research (Fugh-Berman and Scialli, 2006; Sismondo, 2011; Stamatakis et al., 2013). These partnerships therefore suggest an uneven balance of power between corporations and their academic partners, which begs the question: why didn't Unilever suppress the finding that the trans fats in their margarines were hazardous to human health?

However, the assumption that corporations will quash findings that do not accord with their immediate economic interests is based on an exceedingly narrow understanding of organizational rationality. Sociologists have long rejected the notion that individuals or organizations are strictly "rational," i.e. that they only seek to maximize their economic rewards (Smelser, 1998). For example, corporations take political positions based on the personal preferences of senior managers, institutional structures, cultural norms, and organizational learning over time (Hart, 2004). They develop business strategies based not only on financial data but also on instincts, values, trends and best guesses. Financial data is itself based in part on instincts, values, trends and best guesses.

I am not suggesting that corporations do not attempt to protect their interests. I am suggesting that corporations' interests are temporally emergent phenomena. How do corporations' interests change? Rather than always suppressing inconvenient truths, firms also invest in producing scientific research, which they can use as a basis to decide when and how to reorient their interests.

Granted, the second piece of research that I discuss—in which a group of US trade associations and corporations funded research at a government lab specifically in order to disprove Mensink and Katan's findings about trans fats—conforms to the image of industry actors collaborating to discredit scientific findings that contravene their economic interests. The involvement of trade associations in this research is of particular concern, since trade associations have a troubling record of sowing doubt on issues like second-hand tobacco smoke and global warming (Oreskes and Conway, 2010). The industry representatives that I interviewed were themselves scientists and technologists who specified that they chose to collaborate with a USDA researcher in order to get "the best science." When the "best science"—an experiment they had funded, provided materials for and helped to design—also indicated that trans fats increased the risk of heart disease, the resulting claims were credible to the very corporations and trade associations that had collaborated on producing those claims. Industry actors then reoriented their interests around replacing the technology that they had collaborated on turning into a problem. Therefore I argue that collaboration can enhance the credibility of research findings to collaborators themselves.

A Very Useful Fat

Trans fats may have been predisposed to becoming a shared problem in part because so many corporations used or manufactured partially hydrogenated oils. Wilhelm Normann patented the hydrogenation process in 1902. Procter and Gamble bought the patents and commercialized hydrogenation in the United States in 1911 in the form of Crisco shortening. But by 1920, the United States Supreme Court had invalidated Procter and Gamble's patent, arguing in part that shortenings had been a well-established product category long before the development of Crisco (List and Jackson, 2007; List and Jackson, 2009). In fact, the food industry is unique in that its products and technologies are very difficult to patent (Nestle, 2002).

Partial hydrogenation became widespread across the food industry in part because partially hydrogenated oils were very versatile and useful. Soybeans were first farmed commercially in the United States in 1911 (Forrestal, 1982). But the unprocessed oil from soybeans contains fatty acids that oxidize and go rancid very quickly (Dutton, 1951). Partial hydrogenation makes these fatty acids more chemically stable. Partial hydrogenation thus helped create a market for soybean oil. Furthermore, because of their enhanced chemical stability, margarines and other foods made with partial hydrogenated oils have longer shelf lives. Partially hydrogenated oils can remain liquid or can become semi-solid depending on the precise parameters of the hydrogenation reaction. Liquid partially hydrogenated oils burn at fairly high temperatures, meaning they can be used for repeated frying without having to change the oil too often, a costly and messy procedure. Many baked goods can only be made with semi-solid fats. Semi-solid partially hydrogenated oils can be customized with varying plasticities for specific applications in baked goods. By contrast, traditional semi-solid fats like butter, lard and beef tallow have variations in consistency and texture, which is a problem when producing food on industrial scales (Frolich et al., 2014). And unlike animal or dairy fats, vegetable oils like soybean oil are kosher with both meat and dairy products (List et al., 2007).

Because of these advantageous technical properties, partially hydrogenated oils have long been useful to food manufacturers and large food-service operations. In addition, partially hydrogenated oils do not contain saturated fat. Beginning roughly after World War II, nutrition experts, health advocacy organizations and government dietary advice began to associate saturated fats with an increased risk of heart disease, particularly in the United States (La Berge, 2008; Scrinis, 2013). Many of these experts also argued that trans fats were a healthier alternative to saturated fats (Schleifer, 2012). In the late 1980s, after years of advocacy and pressure, many large food manufacturers and restaurant chains, like McDonalds, Burger King, and Frito-Lay, replaced saturated fats such as lard, tallow, palm and coconut oil with partially hydrogenated soybean oil in the late 1980s and early 1990s—and were praised for doing so by CSPI.

Et tu, Margarine?

However, since the 1950s, a few dissenting scientists had argued that trans fats posed a health risk and, in some cases, that saturated fats did not (Johnston et al., 1957; Kummerow, 1986; Enig et al., 1978). This earlier research was often strongly refuted by industry scientists (e.g. Applewhite, 1979). Academic and government scientists often more modestly suggested that trans fats seemed safe, but that further research could help confirm that impression (FASEB, 1976; Dutton, 1979; FASEB, 1985; Kritchevsky, 1983).

Martijn Katan, however, told me that concerns about trans fats were already "stirring" among Dutch nutrition researchers in the 1970s. In the 1970s, the Netherlands Heart Foundation approached him to measure trans fats in commercially available Dutch margarines. He bought margarines in supermarkets, and found that some were free of trans fats but others contained up to 40 percent trans fats. Katan said he had always wondered what effect trans fats could have on cholesterol. But he said that he could not fill in that "nice piece of the puzzle" until Unilever hired a new chief of nutrition named Onno Korver. Katan described Korver as "a very realistic no-tricks person" who, beginning in 1988, "was willing to fund part of our study." According to Kleinman, the questions that academic scientists can ask are limited or even determined by their reliance on materials and tools produced by industry (Kleinman, 2003). But Katan explained to me that all of his trans fat research necessarily involved industry funding or industry materials, because diets containing industrially manufactured foods were his objects of inquiry.

Katan and his assistant Mensink fed human subjects three different diets based on three different types of fats: trans fats, saturated fats, and monounsaturated fats. They fed each subject on each of the three diets in random succession. Katan explained that trans fats are semi-solid or as he put it, "halfway between" between liquid monounsaturated fats and hard saturated fats. He therefore predicted that trans fats would affect "good" HDL cholesterol about "halfway between" the effect on HDL of monounsaturated fats and saturated fats. But he said that their cholesterol measurements "came out totally different from what I had expected and predicted." Their results showed that trans fats lowered HDL cholesterol significantly. "When Ronald Mensink ... showed me that data, my first reaction was 'are you sure this is right?'" He checked to be sure the samples had not been mixed up but "it was just water tight. So it had to be true."

Katan described a friendly relationship with Unilever. As per their agreement, he showed them his results before publication. He said that they too were "surprised" but insisted, "they never tried to maneuver things or influence things or to cover up the observation that trans fatty acids were a lot worse than we had thought up until then." Whereas much of the previous research on trans fats had been published in lipid chemistry or nutrition journals, Mensink and Katan submitted their paper to the *New England Journal of Medicine*, which had not previously published any research on trans fats. Although Katan referred to Unilever as a funder when I interviewed him, the published study acknowledged Unilever only for "developing and manufacturing the special margarines and shortenings" used in the study's experimental diets (Mensink and Katan, 1990). It described the research as "supported by" the Netherlands Nutrition Foundation, the Netherlands Ministry of Welfare, Public Health and Cultural Affairs, the Commission of the European Communities and the Netherlands Heart Foundation.

Before the paper came out, Katan was in Seattle on a brief sabbatical. He said that he received an invitation to dinner from a group of people he described as "the US soybean interests." Recall that most partially hydrogenated fats and oils use soybean oil as a feedstock. Katan told me that the dinner was collegial and convivial until,

> I pulled out the graphs of the *New England* paper which was due to appear in I think one or two weeks. And it became very, very silent. And that showed to me that the data were very convincing. And they were. Because I had made the graphs in such a way that they showed all the individual data. Not just a mean and error bar, but they showed each and every person who had been studied. And it showed you what a lot of subjects there were and how consistent this effect was. So actually I guess some other people were more convinced than I was myself.

While he did not doubt his findings, Katan was concerned that his one study "went so much against what the whole world had believed." He told me that he felt that the editor-in-chief of the *New England Journal of Medicine* had "forced" him to use more definitive language in the article's abstract that he had initially felt was appropriate. The published abstract ultimately stated "The effect of *trans* fatty acids on the serum lipoprotein profile is at least as unfavorable as that of the cholesterol-raising saturated fatty acids, because they not only raise LDL cholesterol levels but also lower HDL cholesterol levels" (Mensink and Katan, 1990). He told me "I was saying I don't want this phrase in. And then they called back maybe half an hour later saying the editor-in-chief had decided that the wording in the abstract had to be 'at least as unfavorable.' That went further than I had wanted it to go. But then who was I to debate the editor-in-chief of the *New England Journal of Medicine*?"

"The main message is to industry"

When Mensink and Katan's study was published, many manufacturing companies had only very recently switched from saturated fats to trans fats, in part due to pressure from activist groups. In April 1990, an activist group called the National Heart Savers Association run by a lone millionaire named Phil Sokolof had purchased full-page advertisements in newspapers including *The New York Times* that praised Kellogg, Sunshine Biscuits, Pepperidge Farms, Quaker Oats, Keebler, General Foods, Pillsbury, Procter and Gamble, Heinz, Ralston Purina, General

Mills and Nabisco for replacing saturated fats with "heart healthy oils," which happened to be partially hydrogenated soybean oil (Sokolof, 1990). Mensink and Katan's study was published four months later.

Immediately before publication, Katan said he worked with Unilever on a press release emphasizing that one study did not justify replacing trans fats with saturated fats in foods—suggesting that Unilever was already concerned that the results of the study would cause consumers or manufacturers to avoid trans fats. Katan said that writing the press release "was all very amicable and serious but it turned out it didn't make a hoot of difference. Because all the US major newspapers and wire services already had the paper three days before we sent out our press release," courtesy of the *New England Journal of Medicine*. Mensink and Katan's collaboration with Unilever did not damage their credibility in the eyes of the US media, which reported their findings widely. The study was on the front pages of *USA Today* and the *San Francisco Chronicle* and in *The New York Times*, *The Washington Post*, *Chicago Tribune* and *Seattle Times* (Friend, 1990; Brody, 1990a; Sugarman, 1990; *The New York Times*, 1990; King, 1990; Brody, 1990b).

Most of the newspapers' stories focused on trans fats in margarine rather than in other packaged foods or in restaurant cooking. Katan reasoned that journalists focused on margarine because they had "been told for years by, say, the American Heart Association, especially by the US scientists that margarines were so much better than butter. And in the US margarines had lots of trans fatty acids." *The New York Times*, for example, stated, "Margarine, the spread millions use instead of butter in hopes of preventing heart disease, contains fatty acids formed during processing that actually increase coronary risk, according to a study published yesterday" (Brody, 1990a). *The New York Times* quoted Scott Grundy, who also wrote an editorial in the *New England Journal of Medicine* accompanying Mensink and Katan's article, saying that "the main message is to industry to provide the public with healthier margarines and shortenings" (Brody, 1990b; Grundy, 1990).

How did "industry" initially respond to this message? Industries are composed of many competing manufacturers, suppliers and intermediaries as well as trade associations. But in this case, a group of firms speaking on behalf of "industry" as a whole responded to Mensink and Katan. The International Food Information Council (IFIC)—an organization supported by food, beverage, and agricultural industries whose mission is to "communicate science-based information on food safety and nutrition" (IFIC, 2009)—responded with a press release the day after *The New York Times* and other newspapers published their articles. The IFIC press release framed the Dutch study as impossible to ignore because it had attracted so much attention from journalists. "Because this question has received broad media coverage, it is important to understand the study in some detail and evaluate its significance to consumers" (IFIC, 1990). It used Katan's own claims to highlight how much the study differed from what was then the more mainstream view of trans fats—and to therefore caution against replacing trans fats. "In announcing the study at a news conference at the University of Washington, Dr Katan emphasized that the results are preliminary and do not warrant changes in current dietary recommendations" (IFIC, 1990). The IFIC press release noted features of the study design that they claimed limited its representativity, including the amounts of trans fats that the human subjects consumed and the amount of time they were given for their serum cholesterol levels to reset between each diet.

The Dutch origin of Mensink and Katan's margarines created an opening for the US food industry to raise doubts about the applicability of their results to American foods. For example, the president of the Institute of Shortening and Edible Oils (ISEO), the trade association that represents edible oil and fat manufacturing firms, wrote a letter to the *New England Journal of Medicine* objecting that the type and amount of trans fats used in the study was atypical of American diets (Reeves, 1991). The ISEO president pointed out that the trans fats in the Dutch margarines were created using isomerization, whereas as the hydrogenation technique is more "typical of the manufacture of U.S. margarine and shortening" (Reeves, 1991). He noted that both isomerization and hydrogenation result in the formation of trans fatty acids with the same types and numbers of atoms in each molecule. But the structural arrangement of atoms on the molecules actually differ, suggesting that their metabolic effects could also differ (Reeves, 1991). He also cited research and reviews that he maintained had established the safety of trans fats, including by the National Academies of Science and the British Nutrition Council (Mattson et al., 1975; British Nutrition Foundation Task Force on Trans Fatty Acids, 1987; National Research Council, 1989; FASEB, 1985; Hunter and Applewhite, 1986).

CSPI initially critiqued the Dutch study on many of the same grounds. Their newsletter included an article based on an interview with a former Procter and Gamble scientist who explained that the isomerization techniques used for creating Dutch margarines differed from the hydrogenation techniques used in the United States (Liebman, 1990). CPSI's article quoted him saying, "'With isomerization, you get a lot of other fatty acids that aren't in our shortenings and margarines,' says Fred Mattson, a hydrogenation expert formerly with Procter and Gamble and the University of California School of Medicine in San Diego" (Liebman, 1990).

J. Edward Hunter, a scientist who identified himself as "from the Procter and Gamble Company" published a book chapter in 1992 making many of the same criticisms of Mensink and Katan's study (1992). Speaking for the edible oil industry as a whole, he was apparently already concerned that the study's findings could precipitate new federal labeling rules and efforts by food manufacturers to replace trans fats. "The edible oil industry believes that the Mensink and Katan study (1990) alone does not provide sufficient justification for major changes in the U.S. dietary recommendations or in the formulation and labeling of food products" (Hunter, 1992). His concerns would prove prescient.

"We have to anticipate the problem"

A professional at a major oil supplier told me that his company's earliest conversations about possible business and health risks associated with trans fats date to 1990. His food manufacturer clients—some of whom had only recently switched from saturated fats to trans fats—began asking him what his solution would be if trans fats became a health issue. "If something becomes a problem then by the time it becomes a problem we need to have a solution. And to do that we have to anticipate the problem and make those investments" he said. In other words, manufacturers were already thinking about switching away from trans fats.

However, a group of industry actors began almost immediately collaborating on research intended to forestall any need to replace trans fats by refuting Mensink and Katan. In fact, I interviewed a consultant who explained that she had worked with various edible oil industry groups for many years. She told me that in order to address Mensink and Katan's study, she brought groups of grocery manufacturers, oil manufacturers, and food product associations together into a group that she called the Trans Fat Coalition. The coalition assembled several consumer products manufacturers, whose names I cannot mention in order to maintain the confidentiality of my interviewees. It also included several trade associations, which are themselves assemblages of otherwise competing firms. These were the American Bakers Association, Grocery Manufacturers of America, Institute of Shortening and Edible Oils, National Association of Margarine Manufacturers, the United Soybean Board (Trans Fat Industry Coalition, 2004; United Soybean Board, 2009). Several of my interviewees indicated that the Trans Fat Coalition started in 1992. Published documents from the United Soybean Board indicate that the Trans Fat Coalition first assembled in April 1994 and continued through 2006, when the FDA's trans fat labeling rule took effect (United Soybean Board, 2009).

The consultant I spoke to emphasized that this type of collaboration is a normal part of how industries operate in the US capital.

> That's been, always in DC, how things operate where you bring trade associations and companies and others together on a common issue where you kind of develop strategies on how to manage an issue, what goes on the communication side and for others doing regulatory work or legislative work, groups like grocery manufacturers and food product associations, others that would have a more direct policy influencing task. So you bring groups together. We talk about an issue. There's been in DC what we call the Trans Fat Coalition. This is a group that has been getting together for probably as long as these issues have been around.

I interviewed several industry professionals who participated in the Trans Fat Coalition. One said emphasized that working across companies allows industries to pool money and set research priorities. He explained that similar groups in the food and oil industries met regularly to "know the science" on specific nutrients like fat, carbohydrates and fiber.

> We look at all these things, trying to find out what's real, what's not. And sometimes it's looking for positive things, what are the positive aspects. Again,

the only thing is that because this is an industry group, we don't share any of our personal stuff, because we're not allowed to. But whatever we can do to work for the betterment of the industry, so that we know the science. Nobody could afford that study by themselves, you know. We don't have that kind of money. But if we get together we can fund some scientific review or scientific research. That's what it's about. And you don't talk business.

Another technologist from a food manufacturing company who was part of the Trans Fat Coalition maintained that Mensink and Katan's study was poorly designed, in part because the concentration of trans fats used in their experimental diet was higher than those in American foods and the isomerization method was different from the hydrogenation method used in the United States. He said, "It wasn't anything like the trans fats the food industry was using. And the food industry thought that it was just a one-off." He said of the Trans Fat Coalition, "It was completely the belief of this group that the Mensink and Katan study was not well done ... and [the Judd study] would show that it wasn't true."

The consultant who led the Trans Fat Coalition explained that organizing the industry around oil was relatively novel because soybean meal, used as a source of protein in animal feed, had traditionally driven soybean sales. Research, innovation and collaboration were therefore usually focused on the protein-rich meal. "Oil was really just an afterthought," she told me. But she said that the Trans Fat Coalition decided they had to conduct their own research on the effects of trans fats. She explained, "The industry itself wanted to get to the bottom on what's going on with trans fat and they spent several millions dollars through USDA in order to get the best science, did a clinical study with Joe Judd." Joseph Judd was a researcher at the USDA's Beltsville Human Nutrition Research Center lab in Maryland. The Beltsville lab, established in the 1890s, is the USDA's oldest human nutrition research laboratory. Judd led a team of five other researchers at Beltsville: Beverly Clevidence, Richard Muesing, Janet Wittes, Matthew Sunkin and John Podczasy.

While Judd and his team were conducting their research, an epidemiologist from Harvard named Walter Willett published an article with his colleagues in *The Lancet* in 1993 that directly associated consumption of trans fats to the risk of heart disease (Willett et al., 1993). Their conclusions were based on data from the Nurses' Health Study. In May 1994, Willett and another colleague wrote an *American Journal of Public Health* editorial estimating that "more than 30000 deaths per year may be due to consumption of partially hydrogenated vegetable fat" (Willett and Ascherio, 1994).

Judd and his team submitted their paper to the *American Journal of Clinical Nutrition* in May 1993. The journal accepted it in October and published it in April 1994 (Judd et al., 1994). But in February 1994, before Judd et al.'s paper was published, CSPI submitted a petition to FDA asking the agency to add trans fats to the newly established Nutrition Facts panels on packaged foods. CSPI's petition cited an in-press copy of Judd's article. The organization was apparently untroubled by the fact that Judd et al.'s study was sponsored by industry—instead acknowledging its industry ties along with the apparent flaws in Mensink and Katan's study. The petition argued, "A study conducted by the United States Department of Agriculture (USDA), sponsored in part by the Institute of Shortening and Edible Oils, is the most definitive of the studies, partly because it tested levels of *trans* (10 grams) similar to those consumed by the average American" (CSPI, 1994).

"Much to the industry's surprise"

The very first line of Judd et al.'s article addressed Mensink and Katan's research:

> In 1990 Mensink and Katan, from the Netherlands, reported that replacement of oleic acid with *trans* unsaturated fatty acid isomers raised low-density-lipoprotein (LDL) cholesterol and lowered high-density-lipoprotein (HDL) cholesterol ... The report by Mensink and Katan raised new concerns with regard to health effects of *trans* fatty acids in the American diet. However, several aspects of the design of the Netherlands study indicated a need for caution in directly extrapolating the results to the American diet. (Judd et al., 1994)

Judd and his coauthors reiterated the critique that the Dutch study had used margarines with concentrations of trans fats that were much higher than was typical of American foods. By contrast, Judd and his coauthors noted that they had used fats supplied by member companies of the Institute of Shortenings and Edible Oils, an American trade association. The study acknowledged funding from food manufacturers and from oil industry, soybean, cottonseed, and food manufacturing trade associations:

> Supported by the Institute of Shortening and Edible Oils, Washington, DC and its member companies; Calsicat Division, Mallinckrodt Specialty Chemicals Company; Illinois Soybean Program Operating Board; Indiana Soybean Development Council; Maryland Soybean Board; Michigan Soybean Promotion Committee; Minnesota Soybean Research and Promotion Council; Nabisco Foods Group; National Association of Margarine Manufacturers; National Cottonseed Products Association; North Carolina Soybean Producers Association; Ohio Soybean Council; Snack Food Association; and United Soybean Board. (Judd et al., 1994)

Judd et al. concluded that trans fats raise LDL cholesterol—the so-called "bad" cholesterol—"to a slightly lesser degree" than saturated fats while also resulting in "minor reductions" of HDL cholesterol, the so-called "good" cholesterol compared with non-hydrogenated vegetable oils (Judd et al., 1994). It concluded, "the present study, together with that of Mensink and Katan and other recent investigations, indicates that dietary *trans* fatty acids may adversely affect plasma cholesterol risk factors for heart disease" (Judd et al., 1994).

The woman who assembled the Trans Fat Coalition told me that Judd and his team's findings had more of an impact on industry than those of Mensink and Katan or Willet and his colleagues. She said Willett et al.'s findings were inherently dubious because they were epidemiological. She maintained that epidemiological studies are "great to develop a hypothesis" but "they don't find dose-response relationships, they don't find a cause and effect." She noted that Judd et al.'s study was a human trial with a significant number of subjects, fed a controlled diet "over a long period of time" in a laboratory setting and assessed for several different physiological indicators of disease risk. She described the Judd team's results as

> the very first really good solid clinical study to show that trans fats—and much to the industry's surprise, nobody thought this was going to happen—but that trans fats may act, if not similarly to saturated fats, but they actually could be a little bit worse because of the HDL factor. The Judd study really was the definitive study.

Nonetheless, she insisted that industry believed the Judd et al. study because of its quality and not because she had her industry collaborators had funded it. "It was the best study, most in depth, and it had nothing to do with the industry funding. It really didn't." Similarly, a trade association representative who was part of the coalition said, "It was the best study that was done to date so that's why everybody was kind of behind Judd. Yes, they were kind of part of funding it but it really was done through USDA with USDA researchers and it was a good clinical study." A trade association official told me his group was doubtful about the validity of the Dutch study. But once Judd et al. showed that trans fats could be risky, he said he had no trouble convincing the corporations represented by his association to support federal labeling of trans fats.

A professional at a food manufacturing company who had been part of the Trans Fat Coalition said that he still had doubts about the results of Judd's team, in part because the concentration of trans fats in the experimental diet was "still too high." Moreover, he was worried about a repeat of the outcry over palm, coconut and other saturated fats in the late 1980s, noting wearily "We wouldn't have been in trans fats if we hadn't gotten out of the tropical oils." He said that the Trans Fat Coalition actually funded further research by the same USDA lab that he referred to as "Judd Two" (Clevidence et al., 1997; Judd et al., 1998).

> The second trial was really well done. I mean the control groups, everything was well done. We worked on it for a year, designing what the study should look like. And I tell you, I was on that design group, and we were looking for good science. We wanted to answer the question, you know, at that point. Because we had gotten negative results from our first one and we needed the answer to the

question. We designed it real well. ... And I think all of us knew when Judd Two came out that trans fats were not what they were thought.

However, by the time those studies came out, it was too late for trans fats. The FDA began to consider CSPI's trans fat labeling petition in 1994. Almost immediately, oilseed trade associations, plant breeders and food manufacturers began working on trans fat replacement technologies (Gupta, 2007; Burton-Cole, 2000). The FDA published is proposed trans fat labeling rule in 1999 (FDA, 1999). Industry actors generally did not dispute the argument that trans fats were harmful to human health. Instead, they supported labeling that would allow them to clearly show to consumers that they had replaced trans fats (Schleifer, 2013).

We Are Our Own Audience

Firms' and industries' economic interests can lead them to defend technologies through practices such as lobbying, marketing and the funding of scientific research. But the trans fat case provides evidence that corporations' and industries' economic interests are not inflexible. How can firms' interests shift such that they replace a technology they previously defended? And beyond individual firms, how can an entire industry decide to abandon a technology? Paradoxically, scientific research initiated in defense of an embattled technology can lead firms and industries to abandon that technology.

On the basis of Mensink and Katan's research, Unilever decided not to defend trans fats. Instead, Unilever worked towards being perceived as a manufacturer of healthier foods by replacing trans fats in its margarines—and then trumpeted its status as a leader in the move towards healthier fats. As Katan and Onno Korver wrote in 2008,

> Unilever aided [Mensink and Katan's] study because the company considered knowledge on trans fats incomplete in spite of their long history of safe use. The decision in 1994 to remove trans fats from Unilever's retail spreads was triggered by media events, but it was built on a solid understanding of the nutritional and technological aspects of trans fats. Over the next 14 years, manufacturers worldwide followed suit. (Korver and Katan, 2008)

The replacement of trans fats that Unilever claims to have initiated is arguably part of a broader trend in the food industry toward developing products that can be labeled and marketed as ostensibly healthier (Schleifer and Desoucey, 2014).

Mensink and Katan's claims apparently convinced Unilever, as well as the editor of the *New England Journal of Medicine*. But the US food and edible oil industry initially rejected Mensink and Katan's claims and initiated research meant to defend trans fats. However, the collaborative nature of this research appears to have initiated an industry-wide shift away from trans fats. Callon has argued that claims gain strength from the heterogeneity of the networks within which they circulate (1991). But the industry collaborators who produced claims about trans fats were both heterogeneous and homogenous. They were heterogeneous in that they represented a range of competing manufacturers, suppliers and trade associations. As a result, the research that they produced was not primarily associated with or stuck inside any one firm. Meanwhile, they were homogenous in that that they all used or produced partially hydrogenated oils, meaning that they all shared an interest in defending trans fats—unless they became convinced that claims about their deleterious effects were credible.

The Trans Fat Coalition members I spoke with said that they were convinced by Judd et al.'s claims because of the inherent quality of the study that produced those claims. But they had designed Judd et al.'s study to meet their criteria of quality by helping to design it and by providing materials and funding. In other words, the producers of the research were also the audience for its results, making those results difficult to dismiss. Maienschein has argued that collaboration can enhance the credibility of scientific claims (1993). By collaborating on the research, these firms and trade associations produced claims that were credible to themselves. They therefore came to see a technology that they had all previously defended as a problem they all shared. As a result, they began to pursue industry-wide efforts to develop and commercialize trans fat alternatives. Changing interests, changing technologies and the near-disappearance of trans fat from the US food system all flowed from corporations' collaboration on research in which they had a vested interest.

References

Angell, S.Y., Silver, L.D., Goldstein, G.P., Johnson, C.M., Deitcher, D.R., Frieden, T.R. and Bassett, M.T. 2009. Cholesterol control beyond the clinic: New York City's trans fat restriction. *Annals of Internal Medicine*, 151, 129–34.

Applewhite, T.H. 1979. Statistical "correlations" relating *trans*-fats to cancer: A commentary. *Federation Proceedings*, 38, 2435.

Berman, E.P. 2012. *Creating the Market University: How Academic Science Became an Economic Engine.* Princeton N.J.: Princeton University Press.

British Nutrition Foundation Task Force on Trans Fatty Acids 1987. *Trans Fatty Acids*. London: British Nutrition Foundation.

Brody, J. 1990a. Margarine, too, is found to have fat that adds to heart risk. *San Francisco Chronicle*, August 16, A1.

Brody, J.E. 1990b. Margarine, too, is found to have the fat that adds to heart risk. *The New York Times*, August 16.

Brouwer, I., Wanders, A.J. and Katan, M.B. 2013. Trans fatty acids and cardiovascular health: Research completed? *European Journal of Clinical Nutrition*, 67, 541–47.

Burton-Cole, J.W. 2000. High-tech soy from back-to-basics breeding. *Agricultural Research*, 48, 23.

Callon, M. 1991. Techno-economic networks and irreversibility. In: Law, J. (ed.) *A Sociology of Monsters: Essays on Power, Technology and Domination.* London: Routledge.

Clevidence, B.A., Judd, J.T., Schaefer, E.J., Jenner, J.L., Lichtenstein, A.H., Muesing, R.A., Wittes, J. and Sunkin, M.E. 1997. Plasma lipoprotein (a) levels in men and women consuming diets enriched in saturated, cis-, or trans-monounsaturated fatty acids. *Arteriosclerosis, Thrombosis and Vascular Biology*, 17, 1657–61.

CSPI 1994. Petition to require trans fatty acids to be combined and labeled together with saturated fatty acids and to prohibit deceptive claims for foods with significant levels of trans fatty acids. Washington, DC: Center for Science in the Public Interest.

Desoucey, M. and Schleifer, D. 2010. Technique and technology in the kitchen: Comparing resistance to municipal trans fat and foie gras bans. *Studies in Law, Politics, and Society*, 51, 185–218.

Doell, D., Folmer, D., Lee, H., Honigfort, M. and Carberry, S. 2012. Updated estimate of trans fat intake by the US population. *Food Additives & Contaminants: Part A*, 29, 861–74.

Dutton, H.J. 1951. The flavor problem of soybean oil. VIII. Linolenic acid. *Journal of the American Oil Chemists' Society*, 28, 115–18.

Dutton, H.J. 1979. Hydrogenation of fats and its significance. In: Emken, E.A. and Dutton, H.J. (eds) *Geometrical and Positional Fatty Acid Isomers.* Champaign, IL: American Oil Chemists' Society.

Enig, M., Munn, R.J. and Keeney, M. 1978. Dietary fat and cancer trends—A critique. *Journal of the Federation of American Societies for Experimental Biology*, 37, 2215–20.

FASEB 1976. Federation of American Societies for Experimental Biology, Life Sciences Research Office Report: Evaluation of the health aspects of hydrogenated soybean oil as a food ingredient. Bethesda, MD and Washington, DC: Prepared for the Food and Drug Administration.

FASEB 1985. Federation of American Societies for Experimental Biology, Life Sciences Research Office Report: Health aspects of dietary trans fatty acids. Senti, F.R. (ed.) Bethesda, Maryland: Prepared for Center for Food Safety and Applied Nutrition, Food and Drug Administration, Department of Health and Human Services.

FDA 1999. Food labeling: Trans fatty acids in nutrition labeling, nutrient content claims, and health claims; Proposed rule. Department of Health and Human Services, Food and Drug Administration.

FDA 2003. Food labeling: Trans fatty acids in nutrition labeling; Consumer research to consider nutrient content and health claims and possible footnote or disclosure statements; Final rule or proposed rule. Department of Health and Human Services, Food and Drug Administration.

FDA 2013a. FDA takes step to further reduce trans fats in processed foods. Department of Health and Human Services, Food and Drug Administration.

FDA 2013b. Tentative determination regarding partially hydrogenated oils; Request for comments and for scientific data and information. *Federal Register.* Department of Health and Human Services, Food and Drug Administration.

Forrestal, D.J. 1982. *The Kernel and the Bean: The 75-Year Story of the Staley Company.* New York: Simon and Schuster.

Friend, T. 1990. Cholesterol: In the spread. *USA Today*, August 16, A1.

Frolich, X., Jauho, M., Penders, B. and Schleifer, D. 2014. Food infrastructures: A preview. *Limn.*

Fugh-Berman, A. and Scialli, A.R. 2006. Gynecologists and estrogen: An affair of the heart. *Perspectives in Biology and Medicine*, 49, 115–30.

Grundy, S.M. 1990. Trans monounsaturated fatty acids and serum cholesterol levels. *New England Journal of Medicine*, 323, 480–81.

Gupta, M.K. 2007. NuSun oil—Success and challenges. *Inform*, 18, 639–41.

Hart, D.M. 2004. "Business" is not an interest group: On the study of companies in American national politics. *Annual Review of Political Science*, 7, 47–69.

Hunter, J.E. 1992. Safety and health effects of isomeric fatty acids. In: Chow, C.K. (ed.) *Fatty Acids in Foods and Their Health Implications.* New York: Marcel Dekker, Inc.

Hunter, J.E. and Applewhite, T.H. 1986. Isomeric fatty acids in the US diet: Levels and health perspectives. *American Journal of Clinical Nutrition*, 44, 707–17.

IFIC 1990. Press release: Hydrogenation of vegetable oils: Perspective on Mensink/Katan study, August 17, 1990. Washington, DC: International Food Information Council.

IFIC 2009. *About the International Food Information Council (IFIC) Foundation*, Washington, DC, http://www.ific.org/about/index.cfm retrieved April 9, 2009.

Institute Of Medicine 1990. *Nutrition Labeling: Issues and Directions for the 1990s*, Washington, DC: National Academy Press.

Institute Of Medicine/National Academies of Science 2005. *Dietary Reference Intakes for Energy, Carbohydrate, Fiber, Fat, Fatty Acids, Cholesterol, Protein, and Amino Acids (Macronutrients)*, Washington, DC, Institute of Medicine and National Academy of Science.

Jacobson, M.F. and Fritschner, S. 1986. *The Fast-Food Guide: What's Good, What's Bad, and How to Tell the Difference.* New York: Workman.

Johnston, P.V., Johnson, O.C. and Kummerow, F.A. 1957. Non-transfer of *trans* fatty acids from mother to young. *Proceedings of the Society for Experimental Biology and Medicine*, 96, 760–62.

Judd, J.T., Baer, D. J., Clevidence, B.A., Muesing, R.A., Chen, S.C., Weststrate, J.A., Meijer, G.W., Wittes, J., Lichtenstein, A.H., Vilella-Bach, M. and Schaefer, E.J. 1998. Effects of margarine compared with those of butter on blood lipid profiles related to cardiovascular disease risk factors in normolipemic adults fed controlled diets. *American Journal of Clinical Nutrition*, 68, 768–77.

Judd, J.T., Clevidence, B.A., Muesing, R.A., Wittes, J., Sunkin, M.E. and Podczasy, J.J. 1994. Dietary trans fatty acids: Effects on plasma lipids and lipoproteins of healthy men and women. *American Journal of Clinical Nutrition*, 59, 861–8.

King, W. 1990. Vegetable oils get some heat as fat-builders—Professor tags "bad" cholesterol. *Seattle Times*, August 16, B3.

Kleinman, D.L. 2003. *Impure Cultures: University Biology and the World of Commerce.* Madison, WI: University of Wisconsin Press.

Korver, O. and Katan, M. 2008. The elimination of trans fats from spreads: How science helped to turn an industry around. *Nutrition Reviews*, 64, 275–9.

Kritchevsky, D. 1983. Influence of *trans* unsaturated fat on experimental atherosclerosis. In: Perkins, E.G. and Visek, W.J. (eds) *Dietary Fats and Health.* Champaign, IL: American Oil Chemists' Society.

Kummerow, F.A. 1986. Dietary effects of trans fatty acids. *Journal of Environmental Pathology, Toxicology and Oncology*, 6, 123–49.

La Berge, A.F. 2008. How the ideology of low fat conquered America. *Journal of the History of Medicine and Allied Sciences*, 63, 139–77.

Liebman, B. 1990. Trans in trouble. *Nutrition Action Healthletter*, 17, 7.

List, G. and Jackson, M.A. 2007. The battle over hydrogenation (1903–1920), Part I: "Crisco vs. Kream-Krisp." *Inform*, 18, 403–5.

List, G. and Jackson, M.A. 2009. The battle over hydrogenation (1903–1920), Part II: Litigation. *Inform*, 20, 395–7.

List, G., Kritchevsky, D. and Ratnayake, W.M.N. 2007. *Trans Fats in Foods.* Urbana, IL: AOCS Press.

Maienschein, J. 1993. Why collaborate? *Journal of the History of Biology*, 26, 167–83.

Mattson, F.H., Hollenbach, E. and Kligman, A. 1975. Effect of hydrogenated fat on the plasma cholesterol and triglyceride levels of man. *American Journal of Clinical Nutrition*, 28, 726–31.

Mensink, R. and Katan, M. 1990. Effect of dietary trans fatty acids on high-density and low-density lipoprotein cholesterol in healthy subjects. *New England Journal of Medicine*, 323, 439–45.

National Research Council 1989. *Diet and Health: Implications for Reducing Chronic Disease Risk.* Washington, DC: National Academy Press.

Nestle, M. 2002. *Food Politics: How the Food Industry Influences Nutrition and Health.* Berkeley: University of California Press.

The New York Times 1990. Margarine's bad side exposed. Study: It's better than butter, but it puts heart at risk. *Chicago Tribune*, August 16.

Oreskes, N. and Conway, E.M. 2010. *Merchants of Doubt: How a Handful of Scientists Obscured the Truth on Issues from Tobacco Smoke to Global Warming.* New York: Bloomsbury Press.

Reeves, R. 1991. Letter to the editor. *New England Journal of Medicine*, 324, 338–9.

Schleifer, D. 2012. The perfect solution: How trans fats became the healthy replacement for saturated fats. *Technology and Culture*, 53, 94–119.

Schleifer, D. 2013. Categories count: Trans fat labeling as a technique of corporate governance. *Social Studies of Science*, 43, 54–77.

Schleifer, D. and Desoucey, M. 2014. What your consumer wants: Business-to-business advertising as a mechanism of market change. *Journal of Cultural Economy*, forthcoming.

Scrinis, G. 2013. *Nutritionism: The Science and Politics of Dietary Advice.* New York: Columbia University Press.

Sismondo, S. 2011. Corporate disguises in medical science: Dodging the interest repertoire. *Bulletin of Science, Technology and Society*, 31, 482–92.

Smelser, N.J. 1998. The rational and the ambivalent in the social sciences. *American Sociological Review*, 63, 1–16.

Sokolof, P. 1990. *The poisoning of America III.* Advertisment in *The New York Times*.

Stamatakis, E., Weiler, R. and Ioannidis, J.P.A. 2013. Undue industry influences that distort healthcare research, strategy, expenditure and practice: A review. *European Journal of Clinical Investigation*, 43, 469–75.

Sugarman, C. 1990. Solid margarine; Heart disease risk linked to certain types of fat. *The Washington Post*, August 28.

Trans Fat Industry Coalition 2004. Letter from the Trans Fat Industry Coalition to FDA on food labeling: Trans fatty acids in nutrition labeling; Consumer research to consider possible footnote statements. FDA Docket 03N-0076 Document C33.

United Soybean Board 2009. *Key activities and major accomplishments: Addressing the trans fat issue 1993–2009.* Chesterfield, MO: United Soybean Board.

Vallas, S.P. and Kleinman, D.L. 2007. Contradiction, convergence and the knowledge economy: The confluence of academic and commercial biotechnology. *Socio-Economic Review*, 6, 283–311.

Willett, W. and Ascherio, A. 1994. Trans fatty acids: Are the effects only marginal? *American Journal of Public Health*, 84, 722–4.

Willett, W., Stampfer, M.J., Manson, J.E., Colditz, G.A., Speizer, F.E., Rosner, D. and Hennekens, C.H. 1993. Intake of trans fatty acids and risk of coronary heart disease among women. *The Lancet*, 341, 581–5.

PART III
Collaborative Health Infrastructures

Chapter 6

The Compound Collaborations of Clinical Registries

Claes-Fredrik Helgesson and Linus Johansson Krafve

Clinical Registries as a Form of Large-Scale Research

The clinical registry constitutes a special form of large-scale research that requires the amassing of data from a large number of patients. The work necessary to make such registries typically involves researchers, nurses, physicians, clinics, and laboratories and centre on the gathering and analysis of observational data of particular kinds of patients. The data aggregated in such registries make it possible to investigate such things as the occurrence of the disease within the aggregated catchment area as well as the distribution of different treatment strategies. A registry normally engages both clinics and care staff not involved in research, and researchers who might be somewhat detached from clinical practice. A registry might, moreover, involve pharmaceutical companies and/or governmental agencies supporting certain parts of the activities related to the registry. Registries thus depend on many different actors and this chapter takes an interest in this particular form of large-scale clinical research by specifically focusing on the diversity and complexity of the many collaborations and interactions involved in the making of such registries. The chapter aims specifically to investigate the collaborations and other forms of interactions related to clinical registries and how these are situated in the large set of institutional ecologies (Star and Griesemer, 1989) that are embedded in sites of clinical care and clinical research.

There are two circumstances that give clinical registries a highly tangled quality. The first circumstance is that clinical registries are by necessity situated in a nexus of research and clinical care. The second circumstance is that clinical registries involve a variety of different actors. Furthermore, each of these actors is regularly involved in other research and care related collaborations and interactions outside the scope of the registry. The tangled quality of a registry is thus related to the variety of research and care-related activities involved, the variety of engaged actors with different orientations, and the many different institutional settings spanned. All this makes it into a compelling research task to examine the diversity and complexity of the many collaborations and interactions that make such a registry possible. It is also pressing to examine how participation in a registry influences other collaborations of involved parties. In this chapter, we address this interest by taking a detailed look at three clinical registries by specifically examining the diversity of collaborations that make up the clinical registries. We also address how participation in the registries influences collaborations within research and clinical practice, outside the scope of the registry. Thus, we approach the three examined registries with the following two questions: What forms of collaborations and interactions make up the registry? How does participation in registry activities relate to other collaborations and interactions in research and clinical practice that enrolled clinics and researchers might be involved in? Our focus on certain relational aspects of clinical registries promises furthermore to provide insight concerning some important conditions for coordination in both clinical research and in clinical practice. At the very least, it can provide insight into the conditions for collaborating and interacting across different institutional settings in clinical care and research.

The outline of the chapter is as follows. The next section introduces some further characteristics of clinical registries and elaborates our focus on collaborations in relation to the registries. The subsequent section introduces a few analytical concepts to aid in the empirical inquiry, along with a note describing our data collection. Next comes a presentation of the three registries examined. The following two sections take on our two research questions, with the first focusing on the collaborations and interactions that *make up* the registries, and the subsequent section focusing on collaborations and interactions that are *associated with*, but not part of, the registries. The concluding section takes stock of the inquiry and particularly focuses on insights regarding the operation of registries and reflects on what this suggests regarding the conditions *for collaboration in clinical research and in clinical practice.*

What a Clinical Registry Is and How It Is Organised

A clinical registry is used for investigating how frequent a disease occurs, differences in treatment strategies, and how patients respond to treatments over time. The results can be published in scientific publications as well as translated into, and used, in clinical guidelines. A central feature of a clinical registry is its *observational* focus, where it gathers data on all patients having a condition within the scope of the given registry. This sets a registry apart from randomised controlled trials (RCTs) where data are collected only for those patients who have been enrolled in the trial according to certain criteria, and where enrolled patients are randomised to receive one of at least two different treatments. A registry, on the other hand, aims to capture data from all relevant patients, and to record their treatments and results. While being a large-scale research endeavour, like RCTs, the data collection of the registry is in some respects more akin to entering information in a patient record. This might best be described as a form for conducting statistical epidemiological research in medicine.

The research endeavours related to registries should also be seen in relation to the increasing emphasis to gain solid scientific evidence for clinical practice. This is often tied to the notion of evidence-based medicine and the idea of fostering more standardised treatment practices based on assessments of the results from large-scale research endeavours (see, for instance, Timmermans and Berg, 2003). RCTs are normally considered to provide more reliable results for such assessments of interventions than are results from observational registries. For our purposes, however, emphasis on scientific evidence means it is important to appreciate that registries are operated in relation to policy, care and research, where assessment and usefulness of clinical research are vibrant topics. In short, registries operate in settings where concerns over what counts as solid and useful knowledge are vibrant matters.

There is a general imperative for clinical registries to include many patients, which translates into a need to bring together patient data from many different clinics seeing the same type of patients. Organisationally, this implies coordinating work to gather similar data from clinics differing in many ways from one another in terms of size, scope of clinical practice, and research orientation (if applicable). Data from different clinics are gathered at an overall registry hub where analysis of data and other general tasks are coordinated, such as the preparation of publications. The research hub is commonly a research-oriented clinic. A registry can, apart from involving different forms of clinics and research centres, also involve other organisations such as professional associations, public agencies, patient organisations, and pharmaceutical industry. A registry can thus span several organisational, national, and professional boundaries and can furthermore engage researchers and clinicians with different orientations.

Conceptualising Relational Aspects of Registries and Their Exploration

The large-scale coordinative quality of registries makes them interesting in relation to the increasing interest in collaboration in life sciences in recent years (for example, Parker et al., 2010, and the current volume). This is, not the least, pertinent given that the registries to some extent carry translational qualities in their recurrent spanning of research and clinical practice (on translational science in medicine, see, for example, Lander and Atkinson-Grosjean, 2011). A registry can in certain matters appear as a single unity, such as in the publishing of guidelines, or a relationally constituted macro-actor (Callon and Latour, 1981; Czarniawska and Hernes, 2005). Our interest in the collaborations and interactions of registries is in this sense an interest in examining the relational constitution of registries as macro-actors.

While it is clear that registries hinge on interactions that span many boundaries, it is not equally clear *how* collaborations and interactions operate within the registries. This concerns, firstly, where coordinated interactions are of such mutual intensity that they can be seen as truly collaborative, and where they are not (see Shrum, 2010). It concerns, secondly, how these interactions are achieved given that they involve parties with different outlooks and positions.

Previously, the notion of 'trading zones' (e.g. Galison, 1999; Gorman, 2010) has been suggested to conceptualise how transgressive collaborations are made possible within the production of scientific knowledge. The trading zone is made up from the coming together of researchers with different outlooks and epistemic orientations in interactions, which in turn create fruitful output. Various forms of interaction and more intense collaboration can thus be seen as taking place in trading zones, where parties of different cultures and orientations meet to 'trade'. Examining how data, knowledge and other 'goods' travel and attain value in different interactions allows us to examine the coordinative operation of the registries.

By using trading zones in the plural we want to avoid presuming that all interactions making up a registry operate according to a single set of rules of engagement. There is quite a substantial literature dealing with these types of rules in terms of the effect of pharmaceutical business on medical research (see, for example, Rasmussen, 2004; Sismondo, 2008; 2009) or more broadly of how collaborations and interactions operate within a distinct moral economy (Kohler, 1994; Daston, 1995). More seldom – and this is where the study aims to make a contribution – trading zones are seen as emergent in practical activities and constructions, which are heterogeneous and enact a multitude of different values, justifications, and purposes that sometimes (but not always) tend to conflict.

Another facet of registries we want to investigate is how they relate to collaborations and interactions outside the scope of the registry. We do this under the proposition that there are *interdependencies* between different collaborations and interactions (see Johanson and Mattsson, 1987) and that these interdependencies can involve activities and actors outside the realm of the registry. The perspective of registries as relational achievements warrants us the possibility not to restrict our view to the interactions that make up the registry, but also to be observant on possible dependencies between collaborations and interactions 'inside' the registry and collaborations and interactions 'outside' the registry.

Our study pursued an exploratory approach where we focused on inter-organisational and financial aspects of the registries. The three registries examined were chosen by the Swedish Medical Products Agency (MPA) since our study was commissioned as part of a larger project at the agency to investigate the operations of registry networks. The MPA project, 'Assessing Drug Effectiveness – Common Opportunities and Challenges for Europe' focussed on registry-based collection of drug treatment data, particularly where multinational data collection is needed, concerning for example orphan diseases. Among the driving forces for these registries are also regulatory requirements imposed upon pharmaceutical companies at the time of approval. The registries examined were thus selected for certain specificities that are not necessarily present in other registries. That said, they share with other large registries the general feature of being constituted by a large number of collaborations and interactions at the centre of the research-care nexus.

Table 6.1   Some basic data about the registries

Registry	SMSreg	Eutos	Eurofever
Disease	Multiple sclerosis	Chronic myeloid leukemia	Auto-inflammatory diseases (primarily among children)
Number of patients (round figure)	12,000	1,000	2,000
Number of clinics	71	n.a.	67
Number of countries	1	14	31
Main registry hub	Stockholm	Heidelberg/ Mannheim and Bologna	Genova
Most important source of financing	The Swedish Association of Local Authorities and Regions (SALAR)	Novartis	European Agency for Health and Consumers (EU)

Sources: LMV report; SMS-reg: Årsberättelse 2009–2010; Eutos: Presentation Hasford at ELN workshop in Mannheim, 1–3 July 2011 (Concerns population-based sub-registry); Eurofever (Toplak et al., 2012).

The empirical material consists primarily of interviews with representatives of the main hubs of each registry as well as representatives of a few centres, usually clinics, participating in each registry. In total, 17 semi-structured interviews with informants based in nine different countries were conducted between March and October 2011.[1] All interviews were recorded and transcribed. The names of informants depicted in quotes are generic Anglo-Saxon pseudonyms to ensure the anonymity of the informants.

We sought to examine different types of clinics to get a picture of how clinician involvement in the registers may vary within each network. The clinic representatives were therefore chosen to allow us to get a picture of how participation in the same registry may look for different types of clinics and in different countries. We have furthermore strived to encounter both research-oriented and less research-oriented centres. However, research-oriented physicians dominate our sample due to our snowballing method for accessing interviewees. All interviews have been entered into a CAQDAS software where they have been coded using primarily a descriptive coding strategy (Saldaña, 2009).

---

1   Representatives from four centres from four different countries were interviewed for Eurofever and representatives from four centres from three different countries were interviewed regarding Eutos. For SMSreg, representatives from three different clinics were interviewed. The interviews ranged from 23m to 2h32m.

Introducing the Registries

The three registries investigated are: SMSreg, a Swedish registry network for multiple sclerosis (MS); Eutos, a European registry network for chronic myeloid leukaemia (CML); and Eurofever, a registry network within paediatric rheumatology collecting information about patients affected by major auto-inflammatory diseases in childhood. Two of the registries are thus pan-European while one is a Swedish network. The table below depicts some key features for each of the three registry networks investigated.

Eurofever is a registry network for collaboration in paediatric rheumatology and concerns auto-inflammatory diseases in childhood. It is a European registry funded with a grant from the European Union and a smaller grant from a pharmaceutical company. Behind the registry, there is a network for clinical trials called Printo. Printo is an international trial organisation that coordinates clinical trials. Eurofever could thus be described as a registry project that emerged through Printo, while it utilises the Printo tool for collecting patient data. The reason to open a registry was the rareness of the diseases. There are about 300 members of Printo, of which 200 are more active. The clinics taking part of Printo are mostly very small and care-oriented, but among the clinics participating in Eurofever there are also those doing research themselves. Several interviewees witness that this therapeutic area is a small world where everybody knows one another.

Working with the Eurofever registry is only a part-time activity for everyone involved, and there is only one full time equivalent allotted to work with administrating the main registry hub. A steering committee consisting of a handful of experts in paediatric diseases is central to registry governance, but there is also a larger meeting once a year where strategic questions are discussed. The first publication with results from the registry was published in 2012 (Toplak et al., 2012). The goal is to keep Eurofever open for a long period, even though the initial grant will soon be terminated. It is difficult to estimate the enrolment rate since the registry is new, but one figure mentioned is that around 100 new patients are entered into the registry each month. Data about an enrolled patient are captured once a year, but the frequency of capture is increased if the patient also is enrolled in a clinical trial related to Printo. Our informants at Eurofever registry centres assert that there can be a substantial time-lag of up to three months from patient visit to submission of data to the registry.

Eutos is a registry for CML, which is a form of leukaemia. It is founded with the support of grants from the European Union, the European Leukemia Net (ELN), and the pharmaceutical company Novartis. Eutos is built up from several regional or national registries within Europe that each collects and administers data from their respective regions. Furthermore, Eutos is partly the result of a professional association, in the sense that it was inspired by the Swedish leukaemia registry, which was run by a professional association of haematologists. However, ELN is an association of physicians, scientists, and patients with interest in leukaemia, rather than a professional association for haematologists. One of the outputs of the registry is an ELN clinical guideline regarding the treatment of CML, published roughly every second year.

Eutos is coordinated from the University of Hiedelberg and it is also where the funding is administered. Novartis is an important funder and cooperates with the clinical side of the Eutos registry. Novartis does not, however, have free access to the data. A part of the payment received from Novartis is on a per patient basis and each completed form delivered to Eutos is reimbursed with 300 Euros from the University of Heidelberg to the national or regional hub delivering the form. In the case of a successful fulfilment of registration, there should be three successive forms, one for each year over a period of three years. It varies, however, whether this reimbursement is passed down further to the clinic seeing the patient and collecting the actual data. Analysis of registry data is conducted by researchers at Munich University.

SMSreg is a Swedish registry only, and thus differs from the other two in being a national instead of an international registry. There is a European version underway, but it has not yet developed into an operational registry. Today, the registry administrator estimates that the registry covers about 11,000 MS patients out of about a total of 17,000 MS patients throughout Sweden. About 1,000 patients are added each year, half of which are recently diagnosed and half of which were previously diagnosed, but have not been in the registry before. There is one full time equivalent salaried to work with the registry; the rest of the work is not refunded.

The major financial support for SMSreg comes from the Swedish Association of Local Authorities and Regions (SALAR), an association for municipalities and county councils in Sweden, of which the latter are responsible for the provision of health care in Sweden. Formally the registry belongs to the Stockholm county council, but in practice it emerged from a professional association of neurologists. The organisation most closely tied to the registry is the MS association, which is detached from other professional bodies. What is particular with the MS association is that it welcomes not only neurologists and other physicians, but also other professionals interested in MS. The governing board of the registry is delegated from the MS association.

Participating clinics are not reimbursed for submitting data to SMSreg. One problem with the registry, mentioned by a representative of the registry, is that there are more data available in the registry than there is capacity to analyse it and use it for publications. There are furthermore several projects conducted with other centres using registry data. There are about 70 clinics submitting data, and 5–10 of these conduct research. But also those clinics not part of the registry are allowed to submit applications to do research on registry data.

The studied registry networks share some important qualities, while they differ in others. They have all built their organisations on similar ideas related to the gathering of large-scale data sets for making analyses for the purposes of research and developing clinical practice. All three registries have an identifiable main registry hub, although this hub might not be geographically distinct, as in the case of Eutos. Usually, researchers and research-oriented clinicians from several participating clinics take part in governing the registry. Governing bodies might, for instance, decide what analyses should be allowed to use the data of the registry.

The organisational structure of the two European registries, Eutos and Eurofever, is more complex than the one of the Swedish *SMSreg*. Eutos and Eurofever can best be characterised as an association of several national and/or regional registries. This heterogeneous basis for Eutos and Eurofever is reflected in significant variations in how work within the respective registries are performed in different clinics. The varying size of patient populations, which relate to differences in incidence for the three different disease areas, is an additional difference between the three registries. Eurofever captures far more rare diseases than the other two.

Recurring parties in the registries are professional associations. SMSreg is directly related to a professional association for researchers and caregivers of MS patients. Eutos is tied to the European Leukaemia Net (ELN), which is an organisation of physicians, scientists, and patients with interest in leukaemia, funded by the European Union. Eurofever, finally, has been promoted by the Autoinflammatory Diseases' Working Group of the Paediatric Rheumatology European Society (PRES), but is also very closely tied to Printo. (We have systematically queried about links between the main registry hub and patient organisations, and can conclude that there indeed are some such connections, but they don't appear to be central to any of the three registries examined.)

Registry networks, such as these investigated here, are thus constituted by a multitude of collaborations and interactions involving hospital clinics, clinics in university hospitals, and clinics that administer regional and international registry centres. There are many roles for involved clinics: they gather and transfer data, and they are more or less involved in the analysis and publication of results based on the data, as well as governing and administering the registry. As will be *highlighted in subsequent sections, these are all significant aspects affecting the possibilities for collaboration for involved actors.*

Exploring Collaborations and Interactions Making Up the Registries

This section explores some of the dyads of collaboration and interaction in making up the registries. This, necessarily incomplete, list focuses on the 'inside' trading zones of collaborations and interactions and how they operate given the varied set of institutional ecologies of clinical care and clinical research. A prime form of dyad is naturally the one between a clinic seeing patients and some form of regional, national, or main registry hub aggregating patient data from several clinics. This principal form of dyad can, as will be depicted below, take many forms. It can be everything from close collaborative forms to infrequent (and maybe somewhat erratic) interactions. Aside from the varied set of collaborations and interactions involving clinics and registry hubs, we furthermore have links to laboratories, pharmaceutical companies as well as professional associations and research agencies. In all, this section aim to illustrate the multifaceted nature of these collaborations and interactions.

The Diversified Dyads: On Connections between Clinics and Registry Hubs

The ways in which patient data are gathered and passed on from clinics varies both within and between the three registries. This is, furthermore, a variation along several dimensions, such as the actual timing and devices used for capturing data and whether these efforts are remunerated. We will here begin to explore the devices and timing for gathering data, and work our way to the matters of compensation and end up looking at the facets of research collaborations within these dyads.

The gathering of data and the registry – clinical practice connection
There is significant variation in how registry data is recorded in relation to the patient visits that give rise to the data. There are some informants maintaining that data regularly are recorded in the registry in direct connection to the patient visit, while others state that registration and reporting take place several weeks after the visit, by relying on entries made in the patient record and similar local deposits. The Swedish SMSreg has the most direct registration and aims to capture data from each visit. The registration is less frequent in the other two registries and there is also a greater delay between patient visit and entering of data. Yet, there is also significant variation in delay of data entry within each registry and, not surprisingly, more so in the larger European ones which in part has grown out of connecting pre-existing regional and national registries.

Timing of registration in relation to the patient visit also ties into whether the registry is perceived as a tool to be used in the actual clinical practice. One idea with the SMSreg is that the registry should be useful in clinical practice, and this should entice physicians to diligently use it for gathering data about their patients. The computer-based registry interface allows a physician to easily retrieve an overview of historical patient data in connection to the patient visit. In clinical practice, then, the registry is enacted almost as a patient record system tailored to the specifics of MS patients. In practice, however, we met both neurologists (those who see MS patients most often) that used the registry in that way, and neurologists who lagged in entering data and therefore found little use of the registry in clinical practice. Moreover, we have indications that the connection between the timely entering of data and its direct use in clinical practice relates to how closely the clinic itself is involved in research or how central MS patients are in the general case-mix of the clinic. It was in the same vein noted that it is less likely that data about patients seeing GPs end up in the registry. (About 10 per cent of all patients see GPs for their MS and this group is underrepresented in the registry.)

The use of aggregated data from the registries at the clinics is also mentioned. Both SMSreg and Eutos allow individual physicians to print overviews of their own patients. However, the individual physician is restricted to see only her own patient data and cannot retrieve and examine other clinicians' data. For clinicians, it is possible to benchmark the results of one's own clinic to the overall result in the registry. The registry hubs wish to have aggregate levels in clinics and county councils available in due time. For now, a registry administrator can pick out certain data sets for comparison when asked for by participating clinics. A more remote link between registry hub and clinical practice is that analyses on registry data might inform clinical practice through the development of guidelines (for an example of a guideline related to ELN, see Baccarani et al., 2013).

The above indicates that there is great variation in the extent to which registries are seen as a directly valuable in clinical practice. Indeed, when discussing the registry in relation to clinical practice, it was far more often discussed as a chore that often had to be set aside when the clinical workload increased:

> So I think in these very rare diseases immediately it doesn't do anything [for clinical practice] … in all honesty it's a chore and one is doing it for the sake of clinical research. (Kelly Clarke, a researcher and physician involved in Eurofever at a university hospital, October 2011)

Moreover, in Eurofever, our informants explained, the lack of time for making the actual registration was typical reason for clinics to not yet having filed data to the registry. Representatives of the main Eurofever registry hub further witnessed very different levels of interest between clinics to participate with patient data. There are to this effect small clinics that participate proportionally more than their bigger counterparts out of interest in the particular diseases. The representatives of the hub also believe that the way the data are filed is variable due to resources within individual clinics.

Repeatedly, managers at main or regional registry hubs express that they have to take different measures to put pressure on clinics to submit their data. Representatives of the main Eurofever hub explain that it is hard work for registry administration to try to get clinics to report their data. So does a representative of a regional Eutos hub, when he explains the difficulties of getting the data into the registry. It takes an awful effort on behalf of the nurse administrator of the registry to call and nag at staff in participating clinics to complete the forms. Moreover, we were by one head of another regional registry hub of Eutos told that he himself had to do such nagging, since delegating it to a junior administrator might mean he would lose friends among his colleagues.

Authorships and financial remuneration for the gathering of data
Clinics involved in gathering data for the registry might be compensated in return for their efforts. The two primary forms of compensations are financial remuneration and the granting of co-authorships on publications based on analysis of registry data. The first publication reporting on the Eurofever registry had for instance 24 persons listed as authors (Toplak et al., 2012). The number of authors

can in some instances even be equated with the number of participating clinics. When we asked how many participating clinics in Eutos there are in Sweden, the informant's response was that there were 28 co-authors in the last submitted paper concerning data from the Nordic countries. Yet, it is a rather common principle to have a threshold number of patients as a requirement for granting authorship, which means that far from all participating clinics are rewarded authorships.

The principles for how to grant authorships are regularly represented in registry regulations. For instance, the Printo bylaws (governing Eurofever) state that the minimum number of patients that must be enrolled to earn an authorship should be determined before the study begins. We have, however, also been informed that there is room for manoeuvre and that granting co-authorships (and ordering them!) is a matter of negotiation and diplomacy:

> Occasionally ... you have experienced that someone was not really happy, then sometimes you think he's right that he's not happy, you say my goodness, I'm sorry, we will, next time we will pay attention and that happens of course too. (Harry Parker, part of team heading Eutos registry network, March 2011)

Another way to compensate for the gathering and submission of patient data is through financial reimbursement. This is most prevalent in Eutos, with its financial backing from Novartis as a critical component, where €300 makes up the payment for a completed form. According to a researcher placed centrally in the ELN, payments are the only way to allow clinics to work with the registry at all. This is a testimony that returns with other informants in Eutos. There are, however, differences as to what extent reimbursements to national or regional hubs within Eutos are passed on to the clinics actually gathering the data. One informant in a regional UK hub at a university hospital said some of the resources were used to pay a data manager, but that some was also passed on to the clinics reporting on their patients. On some occasion, we were learned that payments to a national or regional hub were not passed on to the clinics. In Italy, for instance, the per-patient payment is used to reimburse a central laboratory in order to provide physicians all over the country with free molecular and cytogenetic analysis (for more on this, see below).

Competition and collaboration in the clinic – registry centre connection
The relations between core clinics at university hospitals and the main registry hub contribute to configure the registry as a research collaboration. Researchers from leading research-oriented clinics often populate central governing bodies of the registries, and figure prominently in research publications, and so on. Yet, research is also active in fostering competition. A researcher and physician at a clinic connected to Eurofever in a university hospital mentioned that there is 'friendly competition' between his unit and the main registry hub for Eurofever:

> Yeah. Also there is a, in a way, friendly competition between us and Italy, in Genua [main registry hub]. Because we are the two biggest groups. And of

course we are friends and we depend on each other for collaboration, together we can make a really good product. But you know, in this product we want our brand, you know, well presented. There you go. (Daniel Adams at research-oriented clinic participating in Eurofever, June 2011)

Registry-based research runs the risk of increasing this tension, because its epidemiological focus benefits from good coverage among relevant patients. Researchers in the same area also compete for results and grants. He further explains how they can manage collaboration within the registry by specialising on different research niches:

This is what we decided for [our clinic], yes, the CAPS [one of the diseases in the registry] is not "our core business". Of course we look at the inflammation there and we see how, how is this regulated and how is this seen in other diseases and also you can say, well, you can talk about diseases but you can also talk about techniques. Because we have discussed with other units in Europe, you will focus specifically on that cell, that type of cell, immune, that part of the immune system, I will look outcome from the other way and look on that part of the immune system, and then you can still look at the same disease and be complementary to each other. But it needs a bit of courage and trust also to discuss this with each other. (Daniel Adams at research-oriented clinic participating in Eurofever, June 2011)

There are, in fact, several signs that the competitive tension is not strongest between research-oriented clinics and main registry hub, but tension seems to be more prevalent between research-oriented clinics within the same country. In this case, it is 'because you have to fish in the same pond for grants' to again quote Daniel Adams. A representative of Eutos' main registry hub also confirms that there might be notable issues of competition between researchers from the same country. He exemplifies by mentioning a major European country where such a competitive tension is manifest between clinics participating in the registry. This means, he explains, that representatives of the registry main hub have to be tactful when dealing with the leading researchers and clinics, to keep them all on-board.

Eutos contains an extreme example of tension between participating clinics. In one country in central Europe there are two regional networks. But the two regional hubs do not collaborate with one another, while both report data to the overall Eutos registry. We interviewed the representatives from both of these regional hubs at a Eutos workshop where they participated. The two registries grew up independently, starting from two different clinics. Apparently, the researchers at the two clinics do not collaborate, but both of them collect data in their respective regions and provide them to the European registry. Here, then, they both collaborate with the Eutos main hub, but not with one another. In effect, then, it is the separate connections between the clinics and the main registry hub that allows for pulling together of data, despite competitive tensions between clinics. The central core of the team heading Eutos has, as one of its central member notes, worked together for over 20 years. According to him, other disease areas, such as AML (acute myeloid leukaemia), have failed to establish a European registry precisely because of too intense competition between central research groups.

Another Dyad Making Up the Registries: Relations to the Pharmaceutical Industry

Pharmaceutical companies are another kind of organisation that at times appear to be tied to the registries. This is clearly most marked in the case of Eutos, where Novartis is one of the partners creating the registry. According to a Novartis representative, it could seem peculiar that a pharmaceutical company collaborates in an epidemiologically oriented registry. She claims that there is a general value for her company to understand the pathology of the disease in depth, to know the incidence, available treatment strategies etc., while it doesn't create revenue first-hand. Even though the patent for Novartis in CML treatment is running out, she states that the support for Eutos will not be terminated, because 'we believe in the scientific value of the data'. Whether the data could be used for analysis, and how, is up to the steering committee of Eutos, of which Novartis representatives hold two seats out of 10.

One representative of the Eurofever main registry hub informed us about one pharmaceutical company investing money in the registry. In this case, the registry hub succeeded in receiving support from a major pharmaceutical company interested in one of the rare diseases covered by the registry. Since it is not allowed to use such support to fund anything that the EU grant already covers, support from the company must be earmarked as remuneration to clinics. This support allows remuneration to clinics entering data about patients with that particular disease only. The representative of the main hub stresses, however, that the amount is so low that the clinics are of course not doing it for the money, but that it provides a little something to keep them entering patient data continuously.

Finally, with regards to SMSreg, a representative of the main hub lets us know that it has been deliberately decided not to let pharmaceutical companies into the collaboration. He explains:

> We do not want the registry to be perceived as some sort of control function on behalf of the industry. There was a lot of anxiety about this among the physicians when we started with the registry. We have tried to avoid that connection as far as possible. (Thomas Mason, representative of SMSreg main hub, February 2011)

Both Multifaceted and Diverse Dyads

The above exposé of the central dyads between clinics, registry hubs and pharmaceutical industry brings a highly varied and multifaceted picture. The 'trading' of data for co-authorships and financial compensation, to take two examples, appear in some connections between registry hubs and participating clinics, but not in others. Moreover, the varying presence of such compensations is not correlated to each of the three registries respectively. We have also encountered a great variety of intensity in dyadic interaction. It ranges from rather infrequent interactions and nagging, to more intense collaborations where representatives of a clinic might participate in the governance of the registry.

Our investigation makes us suggest that is helpful to think of each registry as being made up of several trading zones, each operating somewhat differently, if we demand of a trading zone to have distinct characteristics of operation. Even when restricting ourselves to looking only at the dyads between clinics and registry hub, we can distinguish at least two different types of trading zones. One type would then be made of the hub and some research oriented clinics, and is characterised by a certain intensity of collaboration alongside competitive tensions, where co-authorships is a prevalent currency (while not excluding the presence of financial compensations as well). Another type of trading zone would be one of more infrequent interactions and involve clinics that perhaps are not as research oriented or do not focus on the diseases of the registry. In the latter case, co-authorship is not as frequent a currency.

Collaborations and Interactions Associated to the Registry

The previous section explored the 'inside' of the registries through the central dyads that together constitute the registries. It focused on the trading zones of dyadic collaborations and interactions making up the registries. This second part brings attention to how the registries relate to other collaborations and interactions in clinical practice and research. We take interest in the 'outside' of the registries. The question is how participation in registry activities relates to other collaborations and interactions in clinical practice and research?

Facilitating Clinical Collaborations and a Resource in Health Policy Discussions

We have in the previous section touched upon how registries relate to clinical practice: as a supplement to the patient record, as a tool for local overviews, as a developer of guidelines, and indeed as a chore competing for time with clinical practice. All these were instances of how the registry *directly* ties to clinical practice. We here focus on instances where participation in a registry affects other clinically oriented collaborations and interactions.

Several informants relayed that the registry is, for them and their colleagues, a professional network, but with a shifting emphasis on whether it was for the purposes of research and/or clinical development. The latter could be in the form of development of guidelines (see above) but also in form of direct contacts of consultation. The use of the registry to get in contact with other colleagues regarding specific clinical cases was mentioned by participants involved in Eurofever, since the registry concerns a set of very rare diseases which makes it difficult to build a large local body of experience alone. One informant mentions that data from the registry help him understand his own patients' rare diseases. But he also testifies to look at what others have done, and even contacts these physicians.

> You know each other and you can … nowadays with email you can very easily consult each other with clinical problems. (Daniel Adams, physician and researcher at clinic participating in Eurofever, June 2011)

This is an important point, in that the registry becomes a directory, facilitating consultations between physicians that are separated in space. Without the registry, there would be no chance to know where other patients with rare diseases were located and by whom they were treated. This was also stressed by another Eurofever researcher/physician as particularly beneficial for small clinics participating in the registry:

> But, also I think the other thing is for these very small clinics, dealing with patients with very rare and rather difficult diseases, there is the support of the network. There is the idea that you're actually in a network that you got the names of people to email that you can bounce back and forth how you manage them, and that's hugely powerful and that's one of the things that has been built up as part of this, that has probably been for many clinicians the most useful facet, is that actually there's a list of people you email and we had one from, from right down in the Iberian peninsula just before I went on holiday … (Kelly Clarke, heading a national hub in Eurofever registry, October 2011)

Yet another way in which registries matter is in health policy issues. Informants in all three registries mention how data from the registry might be useful to them to influence health policy within their therapeutic area. In particular, this concerns provision of treatment. For instance, a researcher in Sweden involved in Eutos emphasised that data could be used to depict regional variations in treatment patterns. This could be used to highlight which Swedish county councils denied patients good treatment. Another physician and researcher participating in Eurofever gladly talked about registry results as a possible device towards health care bureaucracies in paying for treatments. However, it is not clear to us how often this is used in practice.

One physician and researcher involved in Eutos stresses another quality of the registry and how it is particularly valuable in the context of health management decisions. The registry allows them to answer questions regarding certain patient groups that traditional clinical trials do not ask:

> I think … an additional value of the registry is to explore this tension between what clinical trials are telling us and what's really happening in the wider world. *Because there's this strong tendency for government bodies and financiers to extrapolate*

data from clinical trials. And what we know from clinical trials is ... related to what the statistician has chosen to analyse, and of course what patient went into the clinical trial. So in a clinical trial you just don't have patients over 80, in real life there's a lot of patients over 80 with CML. And in clinical trials you don't have patients who have other serious illnesses: heart disease, stroke, dementia. Is it worth treating those patients? I don't really know because no one knows. (Emphasis added, Daniel Powell, heading a regional hub in Eutos, June 2011)

In these scenarios the registry potentially alters health management decisions, which in turn will affect clinical practice. But we also encountered one example of a reverse connection to health policy. In MS, the introduction of a new pharmaceutical (Tysabri) into the Swedish reimbursement system in 2006 was linked to a requirement that all patients treated with this drug were registered in the SMSreg.

The Registry as Affecting Other Research Collaborations

The other kind of collaborations and interactions we want to consider more closely here are those concerning research. In the previous section we have already depicted how research in these therapeutic areas are characterised by both collaboration and competition. We have, for instance, described how there are competitive tensions in the trading zone where research-oriented clinics and main registry hub collaborate. This subsection focuses on research collaborations and interactions affected by the registries, even though they are outside the scope of the registries.

Registries might relate to other forms of research in connection to multi-centre randomised controlled trials (RCTs). The Eurofever registry, to begin with, actually grew out of such collaboration, and is in effect an extension of a network of trial collaborators. Representatives of the main hub of Eurofever further attest that they sometimes help in establishing contacts between clinics that want to conduct their own research outside of the Eurofever registry. The registry further serves as a platform for clinics to come in contact with pharmaceutical companies to conduct trials, and *vice versa*, it is also a directory for pharmaceutical companies to identify clinics. A representative of the main hub of Eurofever stresses that the registry can play a mediating role in this respect, while they never disclose the identity of patients for recruitment to trials:

> ... let us assume that a company asks if we can identify some patient within the Eurofever to whom we can propose the participation in a clinical trial, we have to say no, because we cannot disclose the name of patients to a pharmaceutical company for a purpose of a trial. So in this case, the link will be indirect, in the sense of, if a company wishes to do a study, they know about Eurofever, ... we can go back to the centres that we know are collecting a particular patient and ask: "Are you willing to consider a participation of your patient to this clinical trial?" (Alfie Booth, representative of Eurofever main hub, March 2011)

The Eutos registry shares with Eurofever the characteristic of having various relations to clinical trials. A part of the Eutos registry, the 'in-study' sub-registry, builds on the follow-up of patients who were enrolled in certain trials involving the Novartis drug Imatinib (patients diagnosed between 2002 and 2006). Yet, the focus is now more on the population-based registry and the Eutos registry does not have as primary objective to be a platform for trials. Data gathered in clinical trials furthermore tend to be much more detailed than data captured by the registry. That said, there are regularly patients in the registry that are also enrolled in RCTs.

Usually, there are no trials based on the SMSreg. Yet, there is currently one trial testing antibodies with the registry as case report form (CRF):

> This is a scientific project run at the Karolinska Institute (KI). The institute has a sponsorship contract with a company to do this project. Data collection is done in the registry. But, the evaluation and monitoring are done by KI staff. So yes and no. The registry has no ties to industry. It is the research group that has received an approval from the registry to do research on the registry. (Thomas Mason, representative of SMSreg main hub, February 2011)

Despite the asserted distance between the registry and industry, it is obvious that it is the registry that enables the collaboration between KI and industry. Yet, the registry and the research institute do not, according to our informant, negotiate contracts that would 'sell out' data.

There are thus several synergies between registries and RCTs. Two of the registries partially grew out of efforts to coordinate trials. The registries, moreover, appear to facilitate the establishment of trials by providing access to clinicians seeing a specific kind of patients, while they can also assist in identifying prospective patients. Whereas patients regularly can only be enrolled in one RCT simultaneously, they can be enrolled in an RCT and one or several registries at the same time. Such double enrolment might, however, give rise to certain precarious issues. A first example of such an issue arises if the trial is double-blind. In such cases, it becomes difficult to enter data about the treatment in the registry form, precisely because this information is blinded during the course of the trial. A second issue that might arise, regardless of whether the trial is blind, is whether the sponsor of the trial – often a pharmaceutical company – allows other patient data to be entered into both the case report form and into the registry. Several informants confirmed that this could become a real issue. Here, the issue is highlighted in discussion with a representative of the MS registry regarding company-sponsored trials, in which patient data are excluded from the registry for the time of the trial:

> Then this becomes a white spot in the registry as you suggest. ... There is in a sense a situation of competition between the trial and the registry. (Thomas Mason, representative of SMSreg main hub, February 2011)

Such blind spots or temporary omissions are, of course, damaging since registries aim to be representative of the patient population. This stands in contrast to trials, where recruited patients are often selected on the basis of certain characteristics. Yet, we have also encountered examples where trial data could be allowed to be accessed for other purposes:

> So we asked Bristol [Bristol-Myers Squibb] if we can use this particular Czech data [from a trial] together with our real live data, and we got a permission. Because it was a phase II trial with no blinding, so, well, it was a contribution of actually patients treated in the frame of clinical trial, however being also registered in our data base. (James Edwards, head of a regional registry hub in Eutos, July 2011)

Registries as Deeply Transgressive and Tangled Endeavours

We take stock of our inquiry into the collaborations and interactions related to clinical registries by way of three broad observations. The first observation concerns the diverse qualities of the collaborations and interactions that make up the registries. All three registries are made up of stronger collaborations between key parties as well as much less intense interactions between registry hubs and more peripheral parties. The stronger collaborations are primarily between selected research-oriented clinics, but include in some instances also a strong connection between the main registry hub and a sponsor. The diversity of dyadic relations for gathering of data is not only apparent in the intensity of interaction, but also in prevalence, and whether this work is reimbursed or compensated. To us, this suggests that it is helpful to think of each registry as being made up of several trading zones, each operating somewhat differently. We do not think that a clinical registry as a collaborative endeavour can be nicely classified with a typology for multi-institutional research collaborations, such as the one proposed by Chompalov and Shrum (1999).

Clinical registries are constituted by linking care to research through the gathering of data. The second observation is that registries are not only made up of a multitude of collaborations and interactions for the purposes of gathering data, but they can create further links within and between research and clinical care. This includes, for instance, the possibility for a clinician to use the registry to get an overview of his or her own patients. Moreover, the registries are associated to other, both research and care-related, collaborations and interactions. The analyses based on registry data can, for instance, provide means to influence health care policy. A registry can furthermore serve as a platform for other collaborative research endeavours. It can facilitate links in care, such as transnational contacts between two physicians each caring for a patient with the same rare disease. Instead of being a form of endeavour that delineates research and clinical care from one another, registries conduit several kinds of links between and within research and care.

The third observation is that registries involve complementarities as well as explicit tensions between involved practices and parties. The work to gather data for a registry is, to take an example of tension, at times referred to as a chore standing in conflict with the everyday demands of clinical practice. In research, leading researchers need to collaborate to ensure good coverage of patient data in the registry, while there are simultaneously competitive tensions where they 'fish in the same pond' for grants. There are, furthermore, tensions that could occur between a registry as a research endeavour and the demands of RCTs involving patients also enrolled in the registry. At the same time, though, there are several professed ways in which clinical practice benefits from a registry and the research it allows. Hence, the registries are imprinted by a dual imperative of collaboration and competition in research.

We can now in a more substantiated way state that clinical registries are deeply tangled endeavours that transgress many institutional ecologies. We would further at this point want to conjecture that the key to the transgressive quality of registries is linked to the diversity of collaborations and interactions that make them up and are associated with them. Indeed, it appears that it is an ordered diversity that holds these transgressive and tangled research endeavours together.

Clinical registries are clearly a special form of large-scale research at the centre of the research-care nexus. They are not unique, however, in the need to transgress different institutional ecologies, since that general need is further felt in many other endeavours in clinical research and care. Here, the case of clinical registries is suggestive that relationally constituted endeavours in the research-care nexus necessitate a variety of collaborations and interactions of different qualities precisely to be able to transgress the different institutional ecologies entailed.

Acknowledgements

Several persons have contributed to this study. A first thanks goes to Nils Feltelius at the Swedish Medical Products Agency. He presented us with the idea to study a set of European disease registries to analyse their working procedures and ability to collect drug effectiveness data and commissioned us to examine the organisational and financial aspects of registry networks. Feltelius further took the initial contacts with the registries that made the subsequent interviews possible, and has also taken great interest in following the subsequent work.

A second thank you goes to our informants. Setting up interviews with those involved in the registries has always been far from easy given their busy schedules. We are therefore very grateful to those who found time to be interviewed and then shared generously their experiences about registries as well as clinical research and clinical practice more broadly.

Finally, we would like to thank the editors and two anonymous reviewers for their helpful comments on previous versions of this chapter.

References

Baccarani, M., Deininger, M., Rosti, G., Hochhaus, A., Soverini, S., Apperley, J., Cervantes, F., et al. 2013. European leukemianet recommendations for the management of chronic myeloid leukemia: 2013. *Blood*, 122(6), 872–84.

Daston, L. 1995. The moral economy of science. *Osiris*, 10, 2–24.

Callon, M. and Latour, B. 1981. Unscrewing the big leviathan: How actors macro-structure reality and how sociologists help them to do so. In: K. Knorr-Cetina and A.V. Cicourel (eds) *Advances in Social Theory and Methodology: Toward an Integration of Micro- and Macro-Sociologies*. London: Routledge and Kegan Paul, 277–303.

Chompalov, I. And Shrum, W. 1999. Institutional collaboration in science: A typology of technological practice. *Science, Technology & Human Values*, 24(3), 338–72.

Czarniawska, B. And Hernes, T. (eds) 2005. *Actor-Network Theory and Organizing*. Copenhagen: Copenhagen Business School Press.

Galison, P. 1999. Trading zone: Coordinating action and belief. In: Biagioli, M. (ed.) *The Science Studies Reader*. New York: Routledge, 137–60.

Gorman, M.E. (ed.) 2010. *Trading Zones and Interactional Expertise*. Cambridge: MIT Press.

Helgesson, C.-F., and Johansson Krafve, L. 2015. Data transfer, values and the holding together of clinical registry networks. In: Dussauge, I., Helgesson, C.-F. and Lee, F. (eds) *Value Practices in the Life Sciences and Medicine*. Oxford: Oxford University Press.

Johanson, J., and Mattsson, L.-G. 1987. Interorganizational relations in industrial systems: A network approach compared with the transaction-cost approach. *International Studies of Management & Organization*, 17(1), 34–48.

Kohler, R.E. 1994. *Lords of the Fly: Drosophila Genetics and the Experimental Life*. Chicago: University of Chicago Press.

Lander, B. and Atkinson-Grosjean, J. 2011. Translational science and the hidden research system in universities and academic hospitals: A case study. *Social Science & Medicine*, 72(4), 537–44.

Rasmussen, N. 2004. The moral economy of the drug company: Medical scientist collaboration in interwar America. *Social Studies of Science*, 34(2), 161–85.

Parker, J.N., Vermeulen, N. and Penders, B. 2010. *Collaboration in the New Life Sciences*. Farnham: Ashgate.

Saldaña, J. 2009. *The Coding Manual for Qualitative Researchers*. Los Angeles: Sage.

Shrum, W. 2010. Collaborationism. In: Parker, John N., Vermeulen, N. and Penders, B. (eds) *Collaboration in the New Life Sciences*. Farnham: Ashgate, 247–58.

Sismondo, S. 2008. How pharmaceutical industry funding affects trial outcomes: Causal structures and responses. *Social Science & Medicine*, 66(9), 1909–14.

Sismondo, S. 2009. Ghosts in the machine. *Social Studies of Science*, 39(2), 171–98.

Star, S.L. and Griesemer, J.R. 1989. Institutional ecology, 'translations' and boundary objects: Amateurs and professionals in Berkeley's Museum of Vertebrate Zoology, 1907–39. *Social Studies of Science*, 19(3), 387–420.

Timmermans, S. and Berg, M. 2003. *The Gold Standard: The Challenge of Evidence-Based Medicine and Standardization in Health Care*. Philadelphia: Temple University Press.

Toplak, N., Frenkel, J., Ozen, S., Lachmann, H.J., Woo, P., Kone-Paut, I., De Benedetti, F., Neven, B., Hofer, M., Dolezalova, P., Kummerle-Deschner, J., Touitou, I., Hentgen, V., Simon, A., Girschick, H., Rose, C., Wouters, C., Vesely, R., Arostegui, J., Stojanov, S., Ozgodan, H., Martini, A., Ruperto, N. and Gattorno, M. 2012. An international registry on autoinflammatory diseases: The Eurofever experience. *Annals of the Rheumatic Diseases,* 71(7), 1177–82.

Chapter 7

Scripted Collaboration: Digitalisation of Care for Children

Inge Lecluijze, Bart Penders, Frans Feron and Klasien Horstman

Introduction

Collaboration and providing care go hand in hand. Care for children is particularly provided in collaborative ways. Deepening expertise and the resulting fragmentation of care practices require more and better collaboration. Collaboration would enable the mixing and matching of expertise and skills to fit the characteristics of any given health care problem. Collaboration to counter fragmentation is receiving a lot of attention from implementation science and health sciences because it is considered conducive to the quality and effectiveness of social, health and clinical care.

More specifically, a lot of attention is being devoted to the role of concrete technologies and innovations meant to improve and stimulate collaboration in health care: clinical pathways, chains of care, multidisciplinary guidelines, electronic patient records and many more. Multidisciplinary and cross-sectoral collaboration has become commonplace in health care as a practice, but also as an object of study and evaluation, critically or otherwise.

A similar trend is visible in care for children and child welfare. Increased professionalisation and rising numbers of service-providing organisations and professionals provide the context for a call for more collaboration (Tonkens, 2008). Dutch child welfare is a continuously changing field in which several collaborative patterns are meant to guarantee quality of care. Next to the 'old' child welfare neighbourhood networks, case consultations and care teams, new forms of collaborations have emerged over recent years. These include youth and family centres and information and communication technology (ICT) infrastructures meant to support collaboration initiatives. This chapter gives a critical sociotechnical analysis of an ICT infrastructure meant to stimulate collaboration in the Dutch field of child welfare: the '*Child Index*'.[1]

The Dutch Child Index is an 'early warning' electronic information infrastructure – an ICT tool – which is intended to stimulate early identification

---

1 We studied the local Dutch Child Index called 'Zorg voor Jeugd' (Care for Youth), which is linked to the national Index 'Verwijsindex Risicojongeren' (Reference Index for Youth at Risk). This chapter uses the term 'Child Index' to refer to the local ICT tool.

of children 'at risk', multidisciplinary collaboration and coordination of care. In practice, the system enables two things. First, professionals can indicate their involvement with a child through a *registration*. Second, professionals can enter a *signal* into the system when they are concerned and consider a child to be 'at risk'. The system does not contain any information regarding the content of the risk, only the fact *that* a child is considered 'at risk'. Signals can refer to a broad spectrum of risks, varying from obesity to criminal behaviour or a neglected appearance. Once two or more signals exist in the system, the Index requires coordination and indicates which organisation should take charge of this task (Zorg voor Jeugd, 2012; cf. Netherlands Youth Institute, 2012).

This new tool allows the 'youth workforce' – the collective of professionals working with youth, including, but not limited to, social workers, school's care coordinators, GPs, child and youth health care physicians and youth psychologists – to exchange information quickly and efficiently. Being aware of each other's involvedness and concerns regarding one specific child should make it easier to collaborate and coordinate care. Policymakers have voiced the expectation that through this system and the ensuing improved collaborations, child welfare will improve and children 'at risk' will get better care sooner.

Since the tragic death of Savanna in 2004, multidisciplinary collaboration has continued to receive increased attention from Dutch policymakers. Savanna was a toddler who was beaten to death by her parents and whose death became a national news item. The incident caused serious debates about collaboration among child welfare professionals. Research showed that the lack of collaboration between the many professionals involved was one of the important factors that contributed to this tragedy (Inspectie Jeugdzorg, 2005). Savanna sadly enough became, and still is, the national representative for the lack of collaboration in Dutch child welfare. To prevent future tragedies, policymakers devised new policies to stimulate and facilitate collaboration among child welfare professionals. Those new policies prominently featured the implementation of novel ICT systems that coached professionals into collaborative working patterns (Van Eijck, 2006; Programmaministerie Jeugd en Gezin, 2007).

Collaboration in child welfare is not new. In 1981, Smith and Hocking already suggested introducing an 'index of concern' to prevent child abuse by improving inter-agency cooperation and coordination. Based on indicators, this instrument would provide professionals a measure of safety and a degree of risk of a child. Since Savanna's death, the topic has been put high on the Dutch policy agenda and has received renewed attention. Despite the fact that child welfare is for all intents and purposes part of public health, sociotechnical analyses of collaborative practices are rare. Nonetheless, child welfare is a very interesting empirical domain in which to study collaboration. Besides the vulnerable population it deals with, it also involves a broad variety of disciplines and organisations with different interests that often work simultaneously to help a single child. A sociotechnical analysis of the Child Index can help us understand the functioning of ICT in collaboration-demanding practices.

The initial goal of the Child Index was to improve collaboration by linking existing digital record systems, collaboration structures and multidisciplinary meetings, and by replacing some of them. We ask whether this new ICT infrastructure lives up to its promises and expectations and stimulates collaboration *in practice*. Developing and introducing a new technology like the Child Index can be considered a process to discipline professionals into desired behaviour; this process can be designed into the new technology. In this view, the Child Index technology can be seen as what Akrich and Latour (1992) called a technological 'script' designed to prescribe professionals' actions and behaviour. Through the Child Index, policymakers and designers intended to discipline professionals into collaborative working patterns. The theoretical notion of scripts is based on the idea that well-designed technological objects can enable or constrain certain actions and behaviours. Analysing the Child Index in terms of scripts enables us to understand the dynamics of these and other technological innovations and enables the study of their practical implications and consequences against the backdrop of their design.

In line with this, we ask to what extent the Child Index script is 'performed' effectively and does indeed coach professionals into collaborative working patterns. We also ask how it prescribes multidisciplinary collaboration in professionals' daily practices and how professionals use the system. Here, we present an empirical analysis of the introduction of the Child Index in Dutch child welfare. It serves as an example of a technical innovation meant to improve multidisciplinary collaboration in the public health domain. First, we will revisit Akrich and Latour's theoretical notion of script and argue that this concept is useful in studying technological innovation processes in child welfare. Second, we will sketch the Child Index's design and which expectations are connected to this tool from the policymakers' and designers' perspective. Subsequently, we will use Akrich and Latour's notion of script to analyse collaboration through the Child Index. Finally, we will discuss which lessons can be drawn regarding the role of the Child Index for collaboration in public youth care and the value of script-based analyses in studying collaboration practices in general.

Technical Objects as 'Scripts'

The introduction of novel technologies is a welcome opportunity to discipline the actions of those engaging with the technology. In the case of child welfare, the attempt to discipline stems from a policy level. According to Akrich (1992) and Akrich and Latour (1992), technical objects incorporate a script that has the potential to prescribe and define users' behaviours and actions. When developing a new technology, designers anticipate the future users' skills, motives, behaviour and interests and use them as raw material to inscribe a desired pattern of behaviour into the new technology. In this way, designers' representations of users and their desired behaviour becomes materialised into a script: the end result of the designers' work. Just like a scenario for a film, this script assigns roles, actions, attributes, relationships, and associations to human and non-human actors (Akrich, 1992).

The notion of a script is central in semiotic approaches to user-technology relations because it studies the incorporation of user representations into a technology. Since these representations lead to design choices that define the future users, designers play an important role in this approach. They aim to shape a new technology in a way that makes people behave alike and that is in accord with the ideal they have in mind. This ideal, or designer vision, is based on hypotheses, predictions, assumptions, and expectations about future users and the world in which the technology is supposed to act. When the envisioned path that a designer wants users to follow is clear, the designers will 'inscribe this vision of the world in the technical content of the new object' (Akrich, 1992: 208). For instance, designers may materially allow or prohibit certain uses or relationships between people and things. A car that can only start when the seat belts are fastened materially prescribes the wearing of seat belts.

Analysing a technology as a script allows us to reveal the ideologies it contains, a process called 'de-scription'. A script-based analysis helps us to understand, describe, identify and explain the translational processes of inscription and description and the roles, actions, attributes, relationships and associations that a script assigns. Hanseth and Monteiro (1997) described script performance through the notion of the strength of an inscription. This strength determines whether users will follow the inscriptions imposed on them and also how easy it is for users to work around the inscriptions. A script is strong when it disciplines its users with little further instructions. It simply forces people to display the intended behaviour or, in Latour's (1991) terminology, the 'program of action'.

The 'European hotel key' (Latour, 1991; 1992) is a classic example used to explain the scripted interaction between technology and society. A hotel manager wanted customers to return hotel keys to the front desk, but noticed that a door sign did not work. A designer charged with the task of developing a technology that prescribed this desired behaviour replaced the sign with a heavy metal weight attached to the keys to remind customers to return them. The key script succeeded because customers executed the intended behaviour. Since they wanted to get rid of the heavy keys before leaving the hotel, they returned them to the front desk.

However, few inscriptions are as successful as the European hotel key. While innovators strive to make people perform an intended behaviour, a script's success depends on what each user does with the inscription. Actors do not always 'subscribe' to the script and perform accordingly. An inscription is a success when the actors collectively perform the script and when their actions fit with those that the script anticipates for them. When users use a technology in alternative ways, this conflicts with the inscribed program of action and they are then following an 'antiprogram' (Akrich and Latour, 1992). For example, you might fasten a car's seat belt, but wear it behind your back. Thus a script's disciplining abilities will always be influenced by the relevance of context and the extent to which a script has to function in varying contexts. Although the hotel key script is very successful, context does still matter. There will always be guests who do not hand in the key at the front desk, because they cannot read a sign or because they do not notice its weight when added to all the other luggage they drag along.

Therefore, Latour (1991) stressed that it is important to follow a technical script and context simultaneously because the social and the technical always interact with and influence each other. This means that when a new technology is introduced, users will reshape the technology and the way in which it may be used because their reactions influence the designers' technology. However, the design of the technology can also constrain the way users relate to the technical object and to each other, so the user and its environment are specified by the introduction of the technology. Because of these relationships it is important for script analysts to go back and forth 'between the designer's *projected user* and the *real user*, between the world inscribed in the object and the world described by its displacement' (Akrich, 1992: 209).

Oudshoorn and Pinch (2003) criticised the script approach for underrepresenting users. Users play an important role in technology development and are actively involved, but the world of designers and technological objects is given more weight in Actor Network Theory (ANT) approaches. The script approach prioritises the agency of designers over the agency of users, so it focuses on designers who are in control while degrading users to objects who can only reject or adopt the script. Therefore, Oudshoorn and Pinch (2003) suggested that the script approach is inadequate for understanding the dynamics of technological innovation. Similarly, Akrich's approach was criticised because it 'tends to neglect the diversity of user groups involved as well as the heterogeneity within these groups' (Oudshoorn et al., 2005: 86).

Despite criticisms, several authors still use the script approach to analyse information technologies in health care settings (Berg, 1997; Winthereik et al., 2008). Oudshoorn et al. (2005) mobilised scripts to conceptualise the connection between the design and use of a new information technology called 'Baby Watch': a video-communication system for watching premature babies in incubators in a neonatology ward. They focused on the distribution of agency and described how a script incorporated in a technology delegates responsibilities, control and agency to the multiple users involved and creates dependencies between them. Furthermore, this study showed how the mismatch between the designers' representations of users and the real users shapes the tool's development and design process. In the 'Baby Watch' example, users' attitudes, reactions, and needs turned out to be different than the designers expected. Initially, only nurses could activate the camera, which made parents dependent on nurses. To remove this restriction, the camera was installed permanently. However, this adjustment changed the delegation of control and responsibilities, which also had unintended effects. When a nurse forgot to remove the camera lid after a medical treatment, parents became anxious.

The script approach was also used by Timmermans and Berg (1997) to study how medical protocols standardise medical work practices. Two protocols (to save patients experiencing cardiac arrest) were analysed as 'technoscientific scripts which crystallise multiple trajectories' (p. 273). They showed that in the process of achieving universality through standardisation, the protocols are changed and re-appropriated. 'Patients and medical personnel are not turned into mindless followers of some pre-set script. On the contrary, seen from their perspectives, it is the protocol's trajectory which is secondary and which is aligned to their own goals and trajectories' (p. 288). Professionals deviated from and tinkered with the protocol in order to make it workable and make it fit pre-existing local infrastructures and the patient's situation.

The abovementioned studies show that script analyses provide fruitful insights into care practices. They show how interactional processes affect technological scripts, the actors involved, collaborative practices and the quality of medical care. Our study adds to this by taking a look at collaboration practices in a specific field of care: *child welfare*. Although closely related to and collaborating with child health care, sociotechnical analyses in this field are rare.

This chapter is about an ICT tool that was introduced in child welfare. Through an empirical analysis of the introduction of the Child Index technology in terms of scripts, we aim to discern the strengths and weaknesses of a script that prescribes professional collaboration through the Child Index and we ask whether the script disciplines and stimulates its users to act and behave in the intended way. In addition to improving our understanding of collaboration and sociotechnical processes in child welfare this way, we also want to use these insights to draw lessons for the health care field.

Methods

This chapter is part of a broader research project that studies the implementation process of the Child Index in practice. Drawing on insights from Science and Technology Studies, the Child Index technology is studied as a sociotechnical trajectory, which implies that we focus on the interaction between science, technology and society. In line with the theoretical notion of the technological script, we study the Child Index as well as its socio-political context.

Taking into account that Oudshoorn and Pinch (2003) stressed the importance of exploring and paying attention to users during new technologies' development and design processes, we 'followed' the introduction of the Child Index in practice as it was planned and performed in a southern province of the Netherlands over four years (between 2009 and 2013). After a brief pilot study, we started our project by doing fieldwork in four municipalities that differ in size, location and the time the introduction of the Index started.

Three ethnographic methods for data collection were used. First, observations provided insight into the world of the Child Index. Inge Lecluijze observed training sessions, steering committee meetings, congresses, preparation activities for an evaluation, chain coordination meetings and a child case meeting. Second, the data collection was followed by analysing relevant documents, websites, newsletters and publications concerning the Child Index, such as intermediary local evaluation reports, policy papers, reports of preceding studies, relevant notes, covenants and articles. Third, data were collected by means of semi-structured interviews with various stakeholders involved with the Child Index (N = 58): policymakers and managers at the municipality level, professionals working at multiple organisations that use the Child Index and employees from organisations that support and facilitate the implementation of the system. Interviewees were recruited via 'snowball sampling' (Atkinson and Flint, 2001).

The in-depth, semi-structured interviews presented several comparable themes to all respondents, including experiences with the Child Index, multidisciplinary collaboration, professional responsibility, chain coordination, privacy, role of parents, process of implementation, role of policy and politics. Interviews lasted from one to two hours and were open enough to accommodate other ideas or go into depth about everyday experiences regarding the Child Index. They were recorded and transcribed ad verbatim with the respondents' permission. A first analysis of the transcripts and field notes was performed through coding in the software program NVivo. While reading and re-reading the transcripts, Inge Lecluijze went through an iterative analysis process that generated new codes as new insights. The attribution of codes and the intermediary results of this process were independently reviewed and refined by all the other authors.

Collaboration through the Child Index: A Script Analysis

Before we show how the youth workforce deals with the Child Index script in practice and to what extent it has a disciplining potential to stimulate collaboration, we will first illustrate the intentions and expectations of the Index's designers and the way their script is introduced in practice.

Scripts at the Drawing Board: The Designers' Perspective

Especially since the dramatic incident with Savanna, the lack of multidisciplinary and inter-organisational collaboration in Dutch child welfare has been considered a major obstacle to preventing problems among Dutch youth. In addition to Savanna, other well-known inquiry reports have also illustrated similar situations in which tragedies occurred while multiple professionals were working with a child without them being aware of each other. The Child Index was designed because policymakers felt the need and responsibility to prevent future tragedies and to counter the lack of collaboration. While the term 'Child Index' refers to the ICT system, for the purpose of this chapter we will use it to include the entire sociotechnical arrangement that is set up to prescribe professionals' actions and to discipline them towards collaboration through the Child Index script.

At the core of the script lies the technical object, the ICT tool itself, which strives to express collaboration in a material way. The system is based upon the idea of linking up or matching professionals' registrations and signals in the system in order to make them aware of each other's involvement and concerns. When two or more professionals are involved with the same child (a 'match'), the system provides a simple overview of whom to contact and collaborate with. The system also automatically generates email messages about the active signals, which are sent to the reporting authorities to provide them with the necessary contact information. Furthermore, the system will automatically appoint a coordinator according to the underlying protocol. An automatic connection can also be built with the organisation's client record system; such a connection can 'feed' the Index by indicating a professional's involvedness with each new client. Finally, to enable and stimulate actual use, the software was designed to be simple and user-friendly.

Complimentary to the material element of the script, the ICT system is also embedded in a specific social and political context that should facilitate a smooth and efficient introduction process. In addition to policy plans, papers, signed covenants and, since 2010, the insertion of a new statutory regulation in the Dutch Youth Care Act, called 'Reference Index for Youth at Risk', that obliges municipalities to 'work' with this new tool, it is also expected that professionals will be disciplined by training sessions, manuals and newsletters. Together, the material and social elements form a sociotechnical arrangement which can be analysed as a script inscribed by designers and indirectly by policymakers. The latter can use this arrangement to express an ideological notion of collaboration and discipline professionals accordingly.

In the design of this arrangement, only a handful of professionals were involved in a local pilot project (cf. Lecluijze et al., 2013). Some professionals were asked to think about the Index's functional design, but only after the basic principles and requirements had been laid down by managers of child welfare organisations. Eventually, 100 professionals from 13 different organisations participated in a four-month pilot project. A project evaluation report concluded that the pilot was successful and that the Child Index was broadly supported by the managers and professionals who participated in the pilot (Nas, 2006). Outside this pilot project, professionals are considered to be users who should use the tool in practice according to the designers' script.

The Child Index users' manual stresses that when professionals use this ICT tool to show their involvement with a child, it will stimulate collaboration and

> the system prevents youngsters from falling between two stools. (Zorg voor Jeugd, 2009)

However, this means that actually using the system – entering registrations or signals – is a prerequisite. The Child Index manual emphasises this by stating:

> it is important that the professionals in the participating organisations actively use the signalling function. (Zorg voor Jeugd, 2009)

Without professionals' input there is no output for professionals: there is no contact information on the screen about possible collaboration partners who have also indicated their involvement or shared risk concerns. It is therefore crucially important to understand how the tool is used in practice and to find out whether and to what extent professionals perform the designers' script and collaborate.

Scripts in Practice: Different Ways to Deal with the Child Index

The designers of the Child Index developed a script for improving collaboration, starting from the idea that the script's design on their drawing board would correspond to performance of this script in practice. We followed the Child Index script in practice, starting from the basic assumption that there is no one-to-one relationship between design and use. Due to the two-way interaction between a script and its users, which is a continuous and dynamic process, the performance of a script never fully corresponds to the way it is designed and intended. However, the extent and the way in which a designers' script is actually performed in practice appears to differ.

Examining the practices of use of the Child Index, we found different degrees of script performance: we distinguish between (1) assimilation, (2) adaptation, (3) rejection, and (4) reconstruction. Within these larger modes of incorporating the Child Index into their daily practice, professionals exhibited a variety of behaviours, highlighting different key elements of the practice they work in. This means that, in practice, each degree of script performance can take shape differently. Although we analytically distinguished between four prominent ways in which professionals deal with the script, empirically those four ways are not mutually exclusive and more ways to deal with the Child Index can be found. Each of the four degrees of script performance will be discussed and supported by illustrative quotes and professionals' explanations.

Assimilation: Adding to the Script

We define assimilation as adopting and incorporating a script into daily professional work practices through additions. While some professionals accept the designers' script, they appear to tailor it to make it workable and to fit their own views and experiences. Especially when a script does not or insufficiently prescribes what the user should do in a certain situation; assimilation fills in the blank spots. Elements are added to the designers' script to clarify it and to make it fit existing work practices and routines. Assimilation of the Child Index takes place in different ways.

A first way to make a script fit work practices is called institutionalisation; it takes place at the organisational level and is mostly initiated by an organisation's management. Future users of the Child Index attend information meetings and training sessions that were developed by the innovators and facilitating organisations. There they receive general written and oral information and instructions on how to use this new tool. Additionally, the former Dutch Ministry of Youth and Family also offered a national booklet and a website with useful criteria for deciding which children are 'at risk' (Meldcriteria.nl, 2010; cf. Keymolen and Broeders, 2011). However, in practice most users still struggle with the following questions: what is an 'at risk' child? How should these risks be assessed in light of the Child Index? And how to determine whether it is necessary to actually enter a signal?

Most organisations anticipated these questions and supplemented the general instructions by formulating an organisational manual, protocol or instruction. These manuals, mostly written by team managers, lay out the procedures and agreements for how to work with the Index. The organisations' aim in adding such manuals to the designers' script was to enable assimilation into the organisational structure and culture. Some manuals aligned the Child Index with existing risk assessment procedures within the organisation:

> Well, within child and youth health care, we use Bakker's Balance Model anyway [...]. Should that lead to the conclusion "signal", [then we] signal. (B1)

Other organisations developed guidelines that included clear definitions professionals can apply:

> There are guidelines for that [...] we have "children who need attention" and "at risk children". [Only] when it really becomes an "at risk child", so actually in case of two or more risk signals, then it must be entered in [the Child Index]. (L2)

Assimilation can also take shape in clarification. This takes place when professionals devise and apply self-developed criteria and definitions to deal with the Child Index in practice. They do this because they consider the designers' script to be unclear or implicit. While many organisations offer their employees manuals with criteria on how and when to use the Index, professionals also use their own definitions and criteria in dealing with the Child Index script. Although trainers instructed professionals that they should make judgements based on their own professional considerations and trust their 'gut feeling' in addition to following the national criteria, one question most frequently occupied professionals' minds and is not easy for them to answer: when do you actually use the Child Index – enter a signal – by registering your name with a child's?

In practice, professionals clarify the script for themselves, leading to a great diversity of criteria. However, professionals also expressed that they find it hard to deal with these individual differences. The current situation around the usage of the Child Index was described as 'every man for himself' (O2), which makes professionals feel uncomfortable and disappointed.

> Yes everyone acts in the way he/she thinks is right. I think that's a shame [...]
> So everybody acts based on their own interpretation. Yes, I do have colleagues

who dutifully register a lot of children in there and I hardly do it. And nobody says a word about it. (O2)

Our empirical analysis also shows that in practice most professionals consciously or unconsciously develop and use their own risk assessment criteria based on their own experiences, views, and context. For example, one of the various criteria that is being applied is based on the seriousness of the risks and a professional's concerns. Some professionals only enter a risk signal when they think a child has serious, severe and/or multiple problems, for example, in cases with suspicions of child abuse.

> So I decided for myself, because I don't have guidelines from my organisation, [to signal] only then, eh, when there really are serious concerns, and for me serious means life threatening. (O2)

In this light, the parents' reactions[2] appear to function as an important criterion as well. In practice, professionals evaluate how parents actually react on the information provided about the Child Index to determine whether it is wise to enter a signal or not.

Additionally, disciplinary backgrounds and practices are used for clarification. Professionals indicate that they use the range of disciplinary services they can offer as a criterion. This means that the Child Index is only used when a professional cannot offer a child enough help on their own and they desire or need help from professionals in other disciplines. A youth physician argued:

> You only use it for those things for which I think that I need others there. (A1)

Disciplinary boundaries also influence professionals' risk assessment criteria. The Child Index script aims at prevention, which means that professionals are supposed to enter all risks or concerns they identify for a child. However, some professionals only work with youth 'at risk' because that is their expertise. They do not enter signals for all the risks they come across. A youth worker explained:

> A signal can be very small yet still generate worries. When, for example, a youngster is smoking dope on the streets every day, that can already be a signal of concern. Actually, I have to report it directly in [the Child Index]. [...] As a youth worker [...] you are always confronted with a lot of problems. (F2)

---

2   Professionals are required to inform parents before entering a signal regarding their child, but professionals consider this to be difficult since parents might not agree with it. The fear that parents will criticise the decision to put their child in the system and might end the relationship with the professional plays a role in professional's considerations regarding use of the system.

That this youth worker has a different definition of a risk then an internal supervisor of a primary school explains the diversity of definitions and criteria applied. All those variations in how and when the Child Index is used puzzle many professionals.

The common feature of institutionalisation and clarification is that both forms of assimilation result in users applying newly formulated criteria and definitions. Besides professionals' needs for clarification and additions to prescribed definitions, a third manifestation of assimilation – collectivisation – results from professionals' need for consultation in using the Index. Collectivisation is performed to deal with a script when consultation and deliberation are insufficiently facilitated by the designers' script. The Child Index script prescribes professionals to use the tool individually, but professionals often choose to do so collectively. The intended individual assessment turns into a deliberative process in practice through which a signal is made common property. The most prominent form of collectivisation takes place when professionals only enter a signal in the Index after having consulted colleagues or other users.

Collective use is not only caused by the pathway of care. Users also prefer to consult others to discuss an 'at risk' child to avoid registering a signal based on an individual consideration. A team manager explained that it is normal in his organisation to have an internal consultation before a signal is registered:

> [W]hen a signal is being entered, they ask me now and then whether it is right or wrong to enter a signal. […] It always goes through me, so I am the central check so to say. […] Then we discuss it together, like what do you want to achieve with your code. (H1)

Such consultations frequently take place in primary and secondary schools. Dutch secondary schools (since 2004) and primary schools (since 2007) work with a School Care and Advice Team, also aiming at multidisciplinary collaboration (ZAT.nl, 2012). Although the professionals on this multidisciplinary team (e.g. a social worker, youth nurse, and the school's internal supervisor) are also potential Index users, this team mostly acts as an 'internal sounding board' (I1) and a first passage point. When a teacher has concerns about a child, the teacher will always first introduce the case to this team for consultation. This implies that collaboration could be started already before Child Index usage is even considered. In turn, this stimulates users' doubts about the added value of the Index.

> In both cases, we discussed it in the care team […] and agreed to report this case at the same time as well. And that's what I did then. […] You are always reporting on behalf of the school. (I1)

As this quote also displays, the existing collaboration structures stimulate professionals to use the Child Index collectively or on behalf of the organisation.

The fact that the Child Index script ties together with several pre-existing internal and external collaboration structures increases collectivisation.

Overall, assimilation is a way for professionals to incorporate the Child Index script into their work practices and to deal with its blank spots. Professionals come up with different criteria and approaches for assessing whether it is wise and necessary to enter a risk signal in the Index; they fill in the blanks themselves. Some professionals go even farther. The next section illustrates that some go against the script, causing variations in how and why the Child Index is used.

Adaptation: Going Against the Script

Another way professionals deal with scripts in practice is through adapting the designers' script. Adaptation takes place when professionals use a script in ways it was not designed and intended to be used. In contrast to assimilation, which is characterised by supplementing the script, adaptation is the result of deviation from the designers' script. In practice, adaptation leads to unintended and unexpected user behaviour because the designers' script is used in an alternative way. Professionals use adaptations when the designers' prescriptions are perceived to be inconvenient, improper or unfeasible. Different kinds of script adaptations can appear in practice, but they share the need or desire to work around the designers' script. Some professionals refer to script adaptations as 'improper use' (H1) of the Index and express their awareness of using the tool in an unintended way. However, using 'workarounds' makes sense to them, given their daily context. Different forms of adaptation can be distinguished.

One frequent used workaround is circumvention. Two professionals perform circumvention when they deliberately create a match in the Child Index by both agreeing to enter a signal. A match is created via oral communication between professionals instead of individual signals that are linked through the system:

> So you agree beforehand, like if you and I just enter a signal, then there will be a match and then at least those parents will be approached by the care provider. (O2)

Agreeing to create a match means that professionals are already aware of each other's involvement when they enter a signal. A prominent reason professionals expressed for doing this is that they want to see a child's situation improved. Purposely creating a match creates a situation in which somebody else, the chain coordinator, becomes responsible for taking action.

In addition to the fact that circumvention is experienced as a safeguard (because professionals expect the created match to make something happen in a case), it is also used out of curiosity and hope. Only through making a match it is possible to find out what will happen when an appointed coordinator takes action and broadens the perspective by involving professionals who have been absent so far:

> [...] Why? Because, of course we know from each other what we bring each other,
> but also to see what will happen then and what the coordination means. (A1)

Another variant of circumvention is inviting others to participate. This is used when the original network of authorised Child Index users is considered to be inadequate. Professionals expand the network through signalling via another authorised professional, causing indirect signals in the Index or inviting authorised or unauthorised professionals who did not previously use the Index to join the actual coordination meeting. One professional described this way of creating matches without interference from the system as acting 'via the backdoor' (oA). Moreover, circumvention is also related to the earlier mentioned collectivisation. Consulting colleagues, verifying intuitions and collaborating are regular tasks in a professional's daily work. Professionals are used to deliberative action when it comes to helping a child and may opt to circumvent the script by using existing collaborative structures, like a case meeting in a Centre for Youth and Family.

Another variant of adaptation that occurs in practice is coercion. Some professionals describe the use of the Child Index as a way to force others involved to do their job and take up their responsibilities with regard to the desired collaboration process.

> Then a signal is entered by us and then they have to do something. So what you
> get is pressure from the system. [...] Actually, that's improper use. (H1)

When professionals adapt the Child Index script in such a way that it becomes a means of coercion, the system functions as a tool for imposing tasks on others, reminding others of their responsibilities, and formalising agreements regarding coordination and collaboration.

Although professionals call this way of using the system 'abuse' or 'improper use', they explain it by pointing to their feelings of helplessness. When inter-organisational consultation and collaboration is desired but does not work out in practice and organisations do not keep their appointments or fulfil their obligations, the Child Index is considered a means to start up action and one of the only ways to mean something for the child. In this light, respondents also mention the covenant all organisations subscribe to, including the decision rules and escalation procedure, and the fact that this covenant is not free of obligations. When organisations do not collaborate, this covenant is something to fall back on and use to put pressure on others. The above mentioned circumvention is also used as means of coercion, because a match created on purpose forces coordinating parties to accept their responsibility and do something for the child:

> [...] at least somebody has to do something. (O2)

Adaptation also exists in the form of closure. Some professionals only use the Index after a child's problems are mapped, when possible collaboration partners are in the picture already and when the usual process for helping a child has been started already.

> To be very honest, for me it's too often a closing entry. In all the busy-ness. [...] I had a couple of times that I couldn't enter it or I couldn't find it, or it didn't work. And then you think, you know what, I'll do that registration some day when I have time. (H2)

Professionals simply forget to use the Child Index because it is not embedded in their daily routines. For instance, it takes too much time or technical problems prevent them from using it. However, since professionals realise that they are supposed to use the Index, they fill it in afterwards to comply with the rules.

In general, adaptation is the result of professionals who adapt and deviate from the designers' script. Going against the Child Index script and creating workarounds leads to unintended script use.

Rejection: Opposition and Non-Use

Besides assimilation and adaptation of scripts, there are also users who do not deal with the script that is offered to them by the designers; they reject the designers' script. Whether and to what extent this rejection takes place depends on users' work practices and characteristics. However, each type of script rejection becomes evident in a form of 'non-use' of the Index in practice. Furthermore, professionals do not only articulate rejection as a way to deal with the Index themselves, but it is also something they frequently observe among other professionals.

One form of script rejection, which is accompanied by a lot of frustration and complaints, is sabotage by other organisations. It points at others who hinder or mess up the designers' script, which leads to wrong use, non-use or partial use of the Child Index script in practice. Sabotage is expressed in several ways. For instance, professionals may notice that some organisations do not complete their Index-related tasks or do not use the Index at all:

> There still are other organisations that deliver care to the child, and we also know that they have concerns and are authorised to use the system, and yet they don't. (F1)

Knowing that some other parties do not use the tool causes doubts about its functioning and also demotivates professionals to perform the Child Index script themselves.

> And others say, yes but when I enter a registration, nobody else registers, while I do know that there are more professionals involved [...] you know, then it is very hard, being an employee, to instinctively keep investing in it over and over again. (F1)

In addition to organisations who do not use the tool, professionals also complain about others that use the Index in a 'wrong' way. In this case, 'wrong' refers to rejection of some script elements which leads to use of the Child Index that is not in accordance with the rules laid down in the covenant. Users are especially frustrated by a lack of communication from the coordinating party and organisations that do not meet their responsibilities.

> When the responsibilities belonging to a coordinating organisation are picked up well, it can work fantastically, I think. But I think that's the place where the hitches do lie at this moment. (I1)

Disappointment and frustration are caused by the fact that other organisations do not live up to the covenant agreements that accompany the designers' script and thus do not meet professionals' expectations regarding proper use of the Index. These negative experiences with sabotage discourage users from following the designers' script themselves and stimulate assimilation, adaptation and, especially, rejection. When professionals expect or notice that nothing happens after they have entered a signal, they often decide to express their concern to an existing physical collaborative network because they do feel the need and responsibility to share their concern.

Whereas sabotage points at other professionals' rejections of script elements, *dismissal* is a form of rejection that professionals practice and decide upon themselves. Users who perform dismissal may reject the designers' script for several reasons, but total non-use is usually a well-considered choice.[3] Most non-users argue that they dismiss the Child Index script and do not use the system because of existing contacts with professionals from other organisations. Professionals explain that finding out whether there are other parties involved and making contact themselves is what they always do; that is a part of their job. Therefore, it often happens that they are already in touch with other organisations to collaborate before they even thought about using the Child Index to indicate their involvedness:

> [...] it has always been my way of working that when I hear at a certain point that there is another organisation involved with that family, then I ask parents whether it is okay if I contact them as well. And then I just look for that contact myself anyway. (G2)

Dismissing the Child Index script does not mean that professionals do not collaborate; they just begin collaboration activities without using the Index as an intermediary. Instead, they create a non-digital match with other parties because

---

3   Wyatt (2003) distinguished between four categories of non-users in a study on Internet use. Dismissal is similar to Wyatt's 'rejecters' category. Additionally, she stressed the possibility of changes in usage patterns due to changes in temporal and social trajectories.

they know through colleagues or parents who is also involved with that particular child. Moreover, some youth workers argue that using the tool would make their job more difficult:

> Actually we don't use it, because together with the youngster you always have to ... yes, you have to report it, or together with the youngster when he/she is older than 18 years [...] Then that relationship of trust is just lost, when you immediately report it. (E2)

Besides, due to a high workload or technical problems (like loss of their password), the Child Index becomes a subordinate part of professionals' working routines. The lack of experience that arises this way creates the feeling that the Index 'is not that much in my system yet' (H2) and 'not alive' (O2).

The abovementioned forms of rejection of the Child Index script are situated and take place in specific contexts. However, they are also influenced by the extent to which organisations assimilate and adapt the designers' script. Assimilation by organisation A can cause rejection of the script by organisation B. For example, when organisation A only signals in case of very serious risks, professionals at organisation B might become non-users because matches rarely appear to occur. The fact that most organisations demonstrate a degree of assimilation, adaptation and rejection creates vicious circles that contribute to professionals complaining about wrong use by others, which stimulates further rejection.

Reconstruction: Users' Active Roles and Ideas

In addition to assimilation, adaptation and rejection, professionals also deal with the Child Index script through reconstruction. Assimilation, adaptation and rejection all create changes and differences in the local performance of a script. Although professionals do not always follow the script (or do so completely) and also change the way they perform the Child Index script to make it fit their day-to-day practice, in those cases there is no form of feedback or interaction with the script's designers. Therefore, those ways of dealing with the script will not lead to formal reconstruction; the script remains as it was designed on the designers' drawing board.

Reconstruction, on the other hand, points at reconfiguration and redesign of the designers' script and results in a revised script. Due to a mutual relationship between designers and users, there is room for interaction, negotiation and mutual feedback. Professionals can provide ideas, proposals and requests drawn from practice that can start formal reconstruction of the designers' script.

Earlier we referred to criticism of the script approach. Oudshoorn and Pinch stressed the dynamics of technological innovation 'where users invent completely new uses and meanings of technologies or where users are actively involved in the design of technologies' (2003: 16). Therefore, they emphasised the important and active role of users in designing scripts. Our empirical analysis confirms this.

Through reconstruction, users try to deal with the Child Index script as active users instead of passive objects.

One form of reconstruction is reconfiguration. Based on their experiences, perspective and context, users articulate how they think the designers' script should be improved in the form of suggestions and proposals. With regard to the Child Index script, all the professionals mentioned a wish for a simplified script. At the same time, according to some professionals, the scope of the Child Index should be broadened. Some, for instance, suggested a new norm: all children and the professionals involved with them should be registered systematically in the Index. If this becomes the new standard, it is expected to increase the acceptance and effectiveness of the tool.

> Yes, I don't think the system is very handy. […] Then I think that at the moment a child is born, it should be registered somewhere, so I can enter a signal against a name. Then it is clear for the whole Netherlands that when you have a child, it will be in an electronic child record somewhere. (O2)

Other professionals only suggested abolishing the manual signalling function based on professionals' considerations of whether a child is at risk. According to those users, automatic registration of all children for whom a request for help is made at a certain organisation should become the new norm. It would make individual considerations unnecessary and acceptance of using the system easier, because information about all the children who receive help would then become digitalised. Moreover, when all children who receive help are in the Child Index along with an overview of all the professionals involved, the tool can also be used to verify information about the number and type of other organisations involved. This wish to be able to consult the Child Index, like a kind of 'logbook' (E2) or 'telephone directory' (L1), was frequently articulated. However, most professionals with a medical background do not support proposals for expanded use or connections with existing medical records, because of their medical treatment relationships and privacy concerns. Other frequently expressed proposals for reconfiguration are: developing new functionalities in the system itself, increasing possibilities to consult other users and extending authorities by linking more organisations to the system.

Despite the active role users try to take through expressing ideas for reconfiguration, actual reconstruction of the designers' script does not take place. Users lack the authority, money or time to reconstruct the designers' script themselves, so those reconfiguration suggestions can be seen as a form of one-sided feedback to the designers. Some of this feedback can eventually lead to reconstruction of the script at the designers' drawing board, but only when it slowly filters through and is picked up by the steering committee and/or designers. However, a lot of feedback never reaches the designers, because there are no formal feedback loops and professionals do not have the means or motivation to fight on the barricades for their ideal Child Index script.

Reconstruction of a script can also take place through redesign. Contrary to the different kinds of assimilation and adaptation, redesign is characterised by an interaction between users and designers. Such a mutual relationship can facilitate feedback and make it possible for designers to redesign a script according to users' needs. However, the script of the Child Index is typically a designers' script and even during the implementation phase there is little interaction between designers and users. In line with this, the possibilities for giving feedback to the Child Index designers are limited and unclear. Some proposals to reconstruct the script appear to reach the steering committee members and do result in concrete changes to the actual design. Examples of script redesign resulted in software changes (e.g. the possibility to mark a signal with an end date, agreements regarding the signals' storing time, removal of classification signals). Besides material changes, redesign also changed the script regarding the number of authorised users. User requests to extend the authority and to add new parties as users expanded the scope of the Index. Although not all suggestions are picked up, this type of reconstruction illustrates that users taking an active role in the development of this script in practice sometimes results in success.

Discussion

From assimilation, adaptation and rejection to reconstruction, professionals display a variety of ways to work with a technology that embodies a technological script that is seemingly unfit for them and their working practice. While the Child Index script is meant to stimulate collaboration across several practices of care for children, it is performed in more creative and variable ways. Users do not subscribe and perform the script in the way policymakers intended and expected and near complete adoption of the designers' script was never observed. Prescribing collaboration, perhaps unsurprisingly, is more complex than making hotel guests return their keys. But why?

When Akrich coined the notion of a script, she used it to provide insight into how designers inscribe new configurations of users into the technical design of a new product during development. Based on how the designer anticipates and defines the competencies and preferences of future users, a technology is developed that aims to discipline users' actions and behaviour. The body of literature she and Latour assembled on scripts and their disciplining characteristics suggests a number of things. First, they argued that the more material a script is via 'technically delegated prescriptions' – and by extension, the fewer accompanying instructions and manuals – the larger and more pervasive its disciplining power would be. It is more difficult to act against material elements in the world than it is to argue with instructions for use (Akrich, 1992). Second, they argued that the distinction between prescriptions and subscriptions is only rendered visible in times of crisis, because then there is a gap between designers' prescriptions and what users subscribe, which enables analysts to retrieve the script.[4] Designers' expectations of users' predetermined competences and things they assimilate – pre-inscriptions – influence the chance for a crisis to appear (Akrich and Latour, 1992).

Interpreting the Child Index along these lines, it becomes clear that the Child Index as a sociotechnical system contains relatively few material elements and many literary companions acting as a guide, guideline or manual. The ability to discipline and coach users into certain behaviours requires a materiality that the Child Index network lacks. Furthermore, the clearly visible distinction between prescriptions and subscriptions of the Child Index points to a crisis. To solve the crisis and narrow the observed gap regarding the Child Index, pre-inscription is required. Pre-inscription is all the work that has to be done before professionals become users. Designers count on earlier distribution of skills among users and bet on a certain predetermination when they develop their prescriptions (Akrich and Latour, 1992; Latour, 1992). Although ICT use and collaboration in child welfare are both pre-inscribed practices, the use of an ICT tool to facilitate multidisciplinary collaboration is new.

Oudshoorn, on the other hand, articulated a broader view of relationships between technologies and users. She criticised Akrich's narrow view of technological development because it only addressed one aspect of configuring the user, namely 'how innovators anticipate the technical competencies and actions of users', and because 'users enter the picture only after a new technology has been introduced' (Oudshoorn 2005: 209). According to Oudshoorn, technological development requires mutual adjustment of both technologies and its users. Therefore, Oudshoorn emphasised the important role of users in technological development.[5] Users are considered to be creative agents who actively engage in configuring their identities. In this view, a technological script will always be affected by its different users in practice due to their active involvement in the innovation process and the co-construction of users and technology.

From this perspective, users (both professionals and especially parents and children) entered the picture too late and were involved too little in the development process. Policymakers used a pilot project to test the designers' script. Although this test was performed in practice, it took place under ideal circumstances. There was enough money, time, and attention, but there were also motivated professionals who had a voice, who were able to express feedback and who were awaiting the Child Index. In general, results and feedback from a pilot project are always based on an ideal situation and not representative of real

---

4   When the distinction is invisible, there is no gap and it is not possible for an analyst to retrieve a script from the situation: to de-scribe a technological object. 'A crisis modifies the direction of the translation from things back to words and allows the analyst to trace the movement from words to things' (Akrich and Latour, 1992: 260).

5   She criticised Akrich because in her approach 'user-technology relations are restricted to technical interactions with the artifacts, thus neglecting the broader cultural dimensions of human agency' (Oudshoorn, 2005: 210).

practice, so a pilot project can never critically test a script. Introducing the Child Index script outside this ideal context affected the script in an unforeseeable way. To enable mutual adjustment and co-construction in such a development process, attention for and involvedness of users are important preconditions. Neglecting human agency and having a one-sided focus on technical interactions hampers 'proper' usage of the Child Index script.

Although Oudshoorn problematised user-technology relationships and gave insight into how these relationships shape design processes, the desirability and feasibility of this new relationship in itself was not questioned. In the context of child welfare and the Child Index, such normative questions should not and cannot be ignored. These normative issues also point to valuable insights into collaboration in care settings.

First, much time and energy was invested to make professionals use the tool in practice. Although the Child Index renewed professionals' attention to multidisciplinary collaboration and improved insight into each other's work practices, the added value of the Index remains doubtful.

Second, professionals articulated the need for analogue spaces and social interactions to be able to collaborate and perform their jobs. Analogue spaces and room for situated considerations are necessary because each child is unique. Professionals change the script because social interaction and non-digital communication are important to them; collaboration is a social affair. Replacing social connections with ICT connections appears to be difficult, and maybe even impossible.

Third, our analysis provides insight into professionals' creativity in dealing with the Child Index script and explains why it is not used as intended. However, the question of whether professionals collaborate is essentially a completely different and more important one than whether they perform the Child Index script. We can show that this particular rendering of collaboration is not subscribed to. However, it is important to realise that not subscribing to the Child Index script does not mean that professionals do not collaborate. They do collaborate with each other in various ways and always try to provide the best possible help for a child. Additionally, child welfare hosts more collaborative initiatives than the Child Index alone. There have always been multiple scripted and unscripted forms and structures of collaboration to provide the best help possible for a child: inter- and intra-organisational case meetings, neighbourhood networks, case consultations at schools and many more.

Is the Child Index an appropriate tool for stimulating collaboration? Especially considering that the domain of child welfare is currently characterised by competition, bureaucracy, and monitoring (Tonkens, 2008). It was and is highly questionable whether children and parents themselves wanted such an ICT tool in the first place. While professionals confirmed the need for improved collaboration, interestingly, professionals who are parent themselves stated that they would not appreciate it if their child was signalled in the Child Index. In particular, families dealing with multiple problems tend to avoid care providers and often do not ask for help themselves. Using the Child Index to signal risks may stimulate this behaviour. Moreover, it remains unclear what effects the Child Index has on the efficiency and amount of collaboration and especially whether and how the signalled child benefits from it.

Collaboration in child welfare, it appears, is not scripted easily. Health care displays a similar trend: due to a focus on deinstitutionalisation, increasing professionalisation requires collaboration and care practices to no longer only take place in medical settings, but to move to home situations. Overall, health care practices are becoming more complex and dispersed. As a response, innovative technologies, like electronic medical records and telecare devices, have been introduced to control and discipline care professionals' behaviour. Technologies prescribing collaboration and sharing information intend to re-couple care practices in order to meet patients' needs. Our analysis shows the complexity of prescribing collaboration in child welfare. The risk of focusing on scripting collaboration in technical ways is to lose sight of actually collaborating and providing care to patients or children in need; that is something worth signalling.

References

Akrich, M. 1992. The description of technological objects. In: W.E. Bijker and J. Law (eds) *Shaping Technology/Building Society*. Cambridge and Massachusetts: MIT Press, 205–24.

Akrich, M. and Latour, B. 1992. A summary of a convenient vocabulary for the semiotics of human and nonhuman assemblies. In: W.E. Bijker and J. Law (eds) *Shaping Technology/Building Society*. Cambridge and Massachusetts: MIT Press, 259–64.

Atkinson, R. and Flint, J. 2001. *Accessing Hidden and Hard-to-Reach Populations: Snowball Research Strategies*, University of Surrey Social Research Update 33, http://sru.soc.surrey.ac.uk/SRU33.html, retrieved 7 October 2012.

Berg, M. 1997. *Rationalizing Medical Work. Decision-Support Techniques and Medical Practices*. Cambridge and Massachusetts: MIT Press.

Eijck, S. Van 2006. *Koersen op. Het kind. Sturingsadvies Deel 1*. Den Haag: Operatie Jong.

Hanseth, O. and Monteiro, E. 1997. Inscribing behaviour in information infrastructure standards. *Accounting, Management and Information Technologies*, 7(4), 183–211.

Inspectie Jeugdzorg 2005. *Onderzoek naar de kwaliteit van het hulpverleningsproces aan S*. Utrecht: Inspectie Jeugdzorg.

Keymolen, E. and Broeders, D. 2011. Innocence lost: Care and control in dutch digital youth care. *British Journal of Social Work*, 1–23.

Latour, B. 1991. Technology is society made durable. In: J. Law (ed.) *A Sociology of Monsters. Essays on Power, Technology and Domination*. London: Routledge, 103–31.

Latour, B. 1992. What are the missing masses? The sociology of a few mundane artifacts. In: W.E. Bijker and J. Law (eds) *Shaping Technology/Building Society: Studies in Sociotechnical Change*. Cambridge and Massachusetts: MIT Press, 225–58.

Lecluijze, I., Penders, B., Feron, F. and Horstman, K. 2013. Innovation and justification in public health: The introduction of the Child Index in the Netherlands. In: D. Strech, I. Hirschberg and G. Marckmann (eds) *Ethics in Public Health and Health Policy. Concepts, Methods, Case studies*. Dordrecht: Springer International, 153–73.

Meldcriteria.nl 2010. *Handreiking voor het melden aan de verwijsindex*. Versie 2.0, http://www.meldcriteria.nl/, retrieved 20 September 2012.

Nas, K. 2006. *Draagvlakonderzoek onder gebruikers Zorg voor Jeugd*. Helmond: Zorg voor Jeugd signaleringssysteem Helmond.

Netherlands Youth Institute 2012. *Youth Policy in the Netherlands*, http://www. youthpolicy.nl/yp/Youth-Policy/Youth-Policy-subjects/Family-and-parenting-support/Family-and-parenting-support-Health-services?highlight=reference, retrieved 25 October 2012.

Oudshoorn, N. and Pinch, T.J. 2003. *How Users Matter. The Co-Construction of Users and Technology*. Massachusetts: MIT Press.

Oudshoorn, N., Brouns, M., and Van Oost, E. 2005. Diversity and distributed agency in the design and use of medical video-communication technologies. In: H. Harbers (ed.) *Inside the Politics of Technology*. Amsterdam: Amsterdam University Press, 85–105.

Programmaministerie Jeugd en Gezin 2007. *Alle kansen voor alle kinderen. Programma voor Jeugd en Gezin 2007–2011*. Den Haag: Programmaministerie Jeugd en Gezin.

Smith, J.I. and Hocking, E. 1981. Index of concern: An instrument for use in treatment of cases of physical abuse of children. *Child Abuse and Neglect*, 5, 275–9.

Timmermans, S. and Berg, M. 1997. Standardization in action: Achieving local universality through medical protocols. *Social Studies of Science*, 27(2): 273–305.

Tonkens, E. 2008. *Mondige Burgers, Getemde Professionals. Marktwerking en Professionaliteit in de Publieke Sector*. Amsterdam: Van Gennep.

Winthereik, B.R., Johannsen, N. And Strand, D.L. 2008. Making technology public. Challenging the notion of script through an e-health demonstration video. *Information Technology & People*, 21(2): 116–32.

Wyatt, S. 2003. Non-users also matter: The construction of users and non-users of the Internet. In: N. Oudshoorn and T.J. Pinch (eds) *How Users Matter. The Co-Construction of Users and Technology*. Massachusetts: MIT Press, 67–79.

ZAT.nl 2012. *Landelijk Steunpunt ZAT*, http://www.zat.nl/eCache/DEF/1/07/486. html, retrieved 18 September 2012.

Zorg voor Jeugd 2009. *Signaleringssysteem Zorg voor Jeugd 3.2. Handleiding signaalgevers*. Zorg voor Jeugd.

Zorg voor Jeugd 2012. *Hoe werkt Zorg voor Jeugd?* http://noord-brabant. zorgvoorjeugd.nu/page.asp?menu_id=55, retrieved 10 October 2012.

PART IV
Collaboration in Health Care

Chapter 8

Shifting Collaborations and the Quest for Legitimacy: Observation of Regenerative Medicine Research in Japan

Koichi Mikami

Introduction

On 12 June 2012, the Japanese Society for Regenerative Medicine (JSRM) held a public lecture in Yokohama, a harbour city about 30 kilometres south of Tokyo, as part of its 11th Annual Congress. The congress was one of the biggest events in the field of regenerative medicine research in several years, not just because it was a once-a-year opportunity for Japanese researchers in this growing field to gather and present their latest achievements but also because it was held consecutively with the annual meeting of the International Society for Stem Cell Research (ISSCR), the international academic society of stem cell scientists. Approximately 800 people attended this two-hour lecture (11th Congress of JSMR, 2012), and I was one of them. In the conference room where the lecture took place, I saw a large number of patients, some of whom were in wheelchairs, their families and caretakers, the recognisable faces of some researchers surrounded by the flocks of businesspeople and many individuals whom I did not recognise and whom possibly the category of 'public' applies to.

The programme of the lecture listed three academic speakers along with a non-academic commentator. Yoshiki Sawa, the chair of this event and also that of the JSRM annual congress, invited the first speaker Shinya Yamanaka, a stem cell scientist known for his reprogramming technique to create induced pluripotent stem (iPS) cells.[1] Yamanaka opened his talk with casual conversation with the chair and the non-academic commentator Takuro Tatsumi – a Japanese actor later revealed to be a senior alumnus of the high school that Yamanaka himself attended – and then explained his future visions of iPS cell research. As soon as he finished his talk he had to leave the room, and the lecture moved on to the second speaker Teruo Okano, a biomedical engineer who developed a technique called 'cell sheet

---

1   Yamanaka invented a technique to induce the similar biological properties to embryonic stem cells to already-differentiated cells of an adult body, creating iPS cells, and for this invention he received the Nobel Prize in 2012.

engineering'[2] and who is also the president of the JSRM. In his presentation, he demonstrated various achievements of his research group and presented his vision of making 'organ factory', which is a manufacturing approach to produce artificial tissues and organs for transplantation therapy. The final speaker was Sawa himself, who is a cardiovascular surgeon renowned for his experiences in heart transplantation. In his talk, three other individuals not listed on the programme approached the stage: they were Sawa's former patients who received 'myoblast cell sheet therapy'[3] for heart disease, invited as panel speakers to comment on their experiences and explain how the therapy improved the quality of their life.

Each of these speakers at this JSRM public lecture, including Sawa's former patients, is appropriate for the main theme of regenerative medicine research in Japan and, given that Yamanaka became the president of the ISSCR after its Yokohama meeting, the selection of the speakers indicated the chair's intention to present 'the state of art' in this research field to the curious public. Yet, this lecture simultaneously embodied 'the state of collaboration' in this field, as each academic speaker has a different disciplinary background, representing a different stance in regenerative medicine research, and, from a social scientist's perspective, the question of why they were all there to speak is worthy of a sociological investigation. Furthermore, the specific audience whom each of them tried to engage also seems reflective of the structure of this research field.

While collaboration in research can be studied at various levels (see Katz and Martin, 1997), in this chapter I examine collaborations in the field of regenerative medicine research in Japan as the configurations of 'clusters', or formal and informal social ties and groupings of different actors. The field of regenerative medicine research is not only interdisciplinary but also argued to lack an agreed-upon definition (Morrison, 2012), and by examining how the clusters have evolved in Japan since 2000, I aim to assess the symbolic significance of the 2012 JSRM lecture for this emerging field. The collaborations in the field are not necessarily directed towards the publication of a scientific article but more likely towards the invention of medical technology, and such collaborations are difficult to assess using bibliometric approaches, as no 'list' of collaborators would be produced in the attainment of this goal (Katz and Martin, 1997). Thus, in my analysis, I draw on the qualitative data collected during five years of sociological fieldwork, including in-depth interviews, reviews of scientific articles and policy documents, and observations at meetings and conferences, all conducted from late 2007 through early 2012.

---

2   Cell sheet engineering is an bio-engineering technique to culture cells in a special petri dish with temperature-responsive polymer coating, which allows researchers to collect cells in a form of a sheet, making it easy to use for both research and therapeutic purposes.

3   Myoblast cell sheet therapy is a clinical application of the abovementioned cell sheet engineering, and myoblast cells obtained from the patient's thigh were cultured as a cell sheet, which was applied to the patient's heart to strengthen its function.

Throughout the chapter, I employ the term 'cluster' to describe social ties and groupings observed in this field for several reasons. Firstly, despite the academic speakers' distinctive disciplinary backgrounds, the term 'cluster' is more fitting than 'discipline' because disciplines are the categories emerged as 'the result of specialization in scientific practice, in terms of the scientific questions pursued and the hypothesis addressed' (Penders et al., 2008: 748). The speakers under this study share practices and visions not only with their fellow scientists but also with many other actors, including funding bodies, corporate partners and even patients and their families. Moreover, the boundaries of clusters are neither self-evident nor fixed, and for this reason even those clustered themselves may not be conscious of their belonging to one or other. As indicated above, the clusters in this field have evolved over the last decade or so, and as such different constituents now than several years ago without them necessarily changing their practices. It is also important to emphasise that while the boundaries of clusters are not evident at the first blush, they are certainly there, and reflecting this point I find the term 'cluster' more appropriate than 'network', which often refers to a linkage of different actors. To refer to what creates the sense of belonging to each cluster, I deploy the word 'style', following Fujimura and Chou's phrase of 'styles of practice', defined as 'historically located and collectively produced work processes, methods and rules for constructing data and theories and verifying theories' (1994: 1017; also cited in Penders et al., 2008). Yet again, I do not limit the use of this term to that of 'scientific' practices and instead apply it to a spectrum of practices and visions involved in regenerative medicine research.

The following sections are ordered nearly chronologically. This study starts in the year 2000, when regenerative medicine research became part of a large-scale, national project in this country. As a result of this turn-of-the-millennium policy initiative, Japanese regenerative medicine research came to resemble 'big science' observed in the latter half of the twentieth century, characterised not only by its volume of funding invested and its number of scientists committed but also by its alignment with non-scientific goals, be it political, economic, or military, and the effort to coordinate different sets of expertise to attain them (e.g. Kelves, 1995; Galison, 1992; Galison and Hevly, 1992). Thus, the year 2000 serves as a reasonable starting point for addressing complex interactions of various actors in this field. As previous studies on research collaboration suggest, becoming 'big science' is not always positive and may come with some costs (e.g. Katz and Martin, 1997; Vermeulen et al., 2010; Weinberg, 1961). Such costs are not only financial, related to the effort of coordinating the collaboration, but also social, associated with the tension arisen within it. While perhaps desirable for maintaining diversity in the field and granting some autonomy to scientists (Vermeulen et al., 2010), the conventional style of small laboratory-based life science research poses significant hurdles for regenerative medicine research in Japan to be coordinated as 'goal-sharing' big science. Therefore, the actors under this study have actively (re-)configured their collaborations so as to achieve legitimacy in this field.

The quest for legitimacy has been a complex process not only because the research field is interdisciplinary but also because of the commitment of the government in the early 2000s rejecting the style of 'pure' science, in which one's scientific legitimacy is achieved by conducting good research and gaining credibility in the scientific community, and instead demanding the shift toward 'clinically relevant' research (cf., Albert and Kleinman, 2011; Bourdieu, 1999; Latour and Woolgar, 1979; Maienschein, 1993). Yet, the cluster of stem cell scientists had difficulties with adjusting their rules and hence changing their styles; biomedical engineers and surgeons, in contrast, came together as another cluster, appreciating the value of patient participation, though it was only possible under a specific legal condition. This situation changed dramatically in 2007 when Yamanaka created human iPS cells, and this event offered a new interpretation of 'clinical relevance'. Having been less successful in its commitment with stem cell science, the government was keen to seize this emerging opportunity and introduced new rules in this field, which again provoked unexpected responses from different research clusters. This Japanese case therefore presents the struggle of shaping a scientific field with the commitment of non-scientific actors, the government in particular. If 'big science' is to be understood as the coordination of research for non-scientific goals (Galison, 1992), then life science research will likely have more of it; yet, as this case shows, there can be a counter move to retain its smallness and hence its purity.

From Stem Cell Science to Regenerative Medicine Research

The new millennium was an important turning point for Japanese science and technology policy. The nation experienced the burst of economic bubble in early 1990s, and little recovery in its economy was observed in its ensuing years (cf., Hayashi and Prescott, 2002). Japan has few natural resources to capitalise on, and hence the government viewed advances in science and technology as promising sources for the nation's recovery, just as they were for the nation's dramatic economic growth in 1970s and 1980s. To promote science and technology within the country, the government enacted the Science and Technology Basic Law and then established the Council of Science and Technology Policy as its internal advisory body in 1995. The Law (1995) stipulates that, upon its consultation with the Council, the government must publish Science and Technology Basic Plans (STBPs) every five years, explicating national strategies for promoting science and technology and also for coordinating plans of related ministries. The first STBP was published in 1996, but this document simply pointed out the need for building national research capacities, suggesting that the size of research population needed to increase and that better research infrastructure ought to be developed (STBP, 1996). It required several more years before the government strategically committed to promoting certain areas of science, and both the Millennium Projects launched in 2000 and the second STBP published in 2001 marked this policy shift.

The Millennium Projects were large-scale government research initiatives focusing on three key themes in modern society – information, ageing and environment. By addressing these themes, research projects were expected to 'resolve the problems that human race would face' and 'result in technological innovation developing new industries' (Kantei, 1999). The government called for research proposals in 1999, and the selected projects commenced in April 2000. As part of the Millennium Genome Project, stem cell science was conducted over five years, corresponding to the theme of ageing. A significant milestone in this national project was the establishment of RIKEN Center for Developmental Biology (CDB) in the harbour city of Kobe in 2000, which has been a key figure in Japanese regenerative medicine research since then. The second STBP (2001) endorsed the visions underlining the Millennium Projects and listed information technology, environmental sciences and life sciences as the national priorities along with five other items. In the section of life sciences, the government clearly stated that it would focus on 'cellular biology, so as to achieve advances in organ transplantation and regenerative medicine' (STBP, 2001: 22–3). Thus, this document officially listed regenerative medicine as an important target for Japan's science and technology.

Enjoying substantial political support for the Millennium Genome Project, Japanese stem cell science made significant progress over the five years of period but its progress was not fully aligned with the original intent of the government. As suggested in the second STBP, the government expected stem cell science to produce 'clinically useful' knowledge, but many research achievements were in animal-based studies on cellular development, differentiation and regeneration. The interim assessment report of the Millennium Genome Project published in 2003 highlighted the need for clear plans to make a transition from basic science to applied research (Kantei, 2003). Like other areas of basic biology, animal cells have been widely used to study biological mechanisms of cellular development, differentiation and regeneration, but, in contrast, human cells, which are critical to understand clinical implications of such mechanisms, were difficult to obtain and only a handful of researchers at university hospitals had access to the cells of donor patients. Despite the significance of RIKEN CDB's location adjunct to a research-focused hospital, stem cell scientists had difficulties with collaborating with medical doctors, who tend to be more interested in improving therapeutic approaches (cf., Cambrosio et al., 2006). The final assessment report published in 2006 stated that the outcomes of stem cell science were 'not ready for clinical applications', leading to the conclusion that the next step was to consider the move into 'translational research' (Kantei, 2006).

Stem cell scientists were not entirely responsible for this mismatch, and the case of human embryonic stem (hES) cell research demonstrates how policy decisions also contributed to it. The growing expectation for stem cell science to make medical innovation at the beginning of the new millennium was partly the result of the establishment of the first hES cell lines by the American scientist James Thomson in 1998. This special type of stem cells has two significant abilities, an ability to be any kind of cells constituting human body and the other to proliferate unlimitedly. These abilities would potentially offer significant advantages for their therapeutic use. However, how nations reacted to these stem cells varied considerably due to the ethical concerns about their research use (Gottweis et al., 2009). The US government announced in 2001 that the National Institutes of Health would only support hES cell research using already established cell lines, and in contrast the UK government authorised research on hES cells for the purpose of developing new treatments under its Human Fertilisation and Embryology (Research Purposes) Regulation 2001. In the same year, the Japanese Ministry of Education, Culture, Sports, Science and Technology (MEXT) also manifested its attitude toward these cells in its Guidelines for Derivation and Utilization of Human Embryonic Stem Cells.

The Guidelines (2001) did not ban hES cell research but rather made it difficult to undertake it in Japan particularly for two reasons. Firstly, the Guidelines stated that 'a human embryo is a beginning of life' and that 'human ES cells have the potential to differentiate into any types of human cells' (2001: Article 3). Following this idea, the Guidelines required both derivation and use of hES cells to pass a dual review process: firstly by the institutional review board of one's organisation and then by the Ministry, thereby rendering hES cell research both labour-intensive and time-consuming. Secondly, the Guidelines undermined the 'therapeutic promise' of hES cells – limiting the need for hES cell research in Japan and rejecting the powerful argument for making hES cell available for research in some other countries (cf., Rubin, 2008). By stating that 'clinical research applying human ES cells or cells originated from them to the human body, and utilization of them in medicine and in its related fields' ought not to be carried out 'until specific criteria other than the Guidelines have been established' (2001: Article 2.2), they caused great uncertainty over medical significance of these cells. This policy decision discouraged the researchers to conduct hES cell research. As a result, Japanese stem cell science progressed without much action in hES cell research (Nakatsuji, 2007), and many researchers chose to study mouse ES cells for their basic research, which exhibit fewer ethical concerns and have been available for long time. Thus, the Guidelines enlarged the gap between basic and applied research in stem cell science.

In accordance with the original STBP policy vision of promoting the production of clinically useful knowledge, MEXT decided to push other areas of stem cell science towards a more clinical orientation, rather than overturning its decision on hES cell research, and launched the 'Project for Realization of Regenerative Medicine' in 2003. As its title shows, this project was designed to focus on clinical applications of stem cells, and the two of its three principal investigators were based at university hospitals, encouraging the kind of collaboration that the Millennium Genome Project was not successful to initiate. Yet, the project leader and the third principal figure were nominated from RIKEN CDB and hence the project was complementary to stem cell science in the Millennium Genome Project, which ended in 2005. Among various non-hES cells, mesenchymal and haematopoietic stem cells in particular were considered to be promising sources for regenerative medicine in this project, and this led to the establishment of a cord blood stem cell bank. This bank was expected to provide stem cell scientists with easy access to ethically-sourced human multipotent stem cells, just as the UK Stem Cell Bank was designed for hES cells (Stephens et al., 2008). This project ran its first term for five years, and it was in its fifth and final year when Yanamaka's research group announced its creation of human iPS cells – an innovation that dramatically changed the state of Japanese regenerative medicine research.

Collaborations at University Hospitals

While MEXT struggled to let stem cell scientists work on human cells, several other actors were actively working on them already, and the works of Teruo Okano and Yoshiki Sawa illuminates this side of the field. Okano developed the abovementioned 'cell sheet engineering' technique in the mid-1990s. When cells are cultured in a petri dish, usually an enzyme needs to be applied to isolate them for collection but its application also causes some damage to the cells. To resolve this problem, Okano invented a special petri dish with temperature-responsive polymer coating: this invention allows the cultured cells to be collected in the form of a sheet simply by changing its temperature without causing any damage (Okano et al., 1995). The cell sheet removed from the petri dish can also be applied directly onto the site of the body in need of therapy, rather than releasing the cells into the body by injection. This new approach is expected to be more effective for therapy because most cells stay at the intended site and perform their functions, while the injection approach must depend on body's biological mechanisms to guide the cells to the deformed site.

Okano not only developed this technique but also promoted its clinical applications actively. In 2001, he established a spin-off company to make his petri dish available for research use. Based at a medial university, his research group also teamed up with surgeons and initiated clinical research using the technique. Once he began such research, some medical doctors from other university hospitals became interested in collaborating with his group. The early successes of such collaborations were on cornea and heart therapies. Severe corneal diseases can be treated by transplantation and this is a well-established medical practice, but the scarcity of corneal tissues for transplantation has been a major challenge. Okano's technique allows a doctor to culture the cells obtained from a patient's mouth in the form of a sheet, which can be transplanted back to the patient's cornea, rather than depending on cornea donation. Similarly, cells procured from a patient's thigh can be used to produce cell sheets, which are then applied to the heart to treat heart failure. This is an attractive alternative to heart transplantation in Japan, where cadaver donors are scarce for its socio-historical reasons (cf., Lock, 2002). Yoshiki Sawa was one of Okano's main collaborators for this myoblast cell sheet therapy, and in fact the patients spoke in the 2012 JSRM public lecture were the first recipients of this therapy as part of the clinical research jointly conducted by Okano and Sawa.

These clinical studies of cell sheet therapies represent a different research cluster of regenerative medicine in Japan from that of stem cell science. They focused on adult somatic cells, which are already differentiated into certain lineages of cellular development, and mainly dealt with their structural matrices, rather than the mechanisms of cell expansion and differentiation. The style of their practice was goal-oriented, which is stereotypic of engineering and medical sciences. This is not to suggest that all collaborators in this cluster shared a single goal. Instead, each of these actors had a personal goal and in order to attain it, collaboration was critical: while Okano, the biomedical engineer, had the special petri dish, he needed access to both the patients and their cells to prove the value of his invention as a tool for regenerative medicine. In contrast, Sawa, the surgeon, needed the petri dish and the skills in culturing cells to treat his seriously-ill patients, as donated organs were unlikely to be available for transplantation. Moreover, because this yet-to-be-approved therapy must be conducted as clinical research, the patients needed the surgeon and his authority in medicine to take part in it.

In this collaboration, each of the actors also had something to offer to the others. The biomedical engineer offered his petri dish, the patients their cells. While these two items are material components of this regenerative medicine approach, the space within a hospital, which only the surgeon could provide, was indispensable for making their collaboration. Until 2006, no guidelines on clinical research using human cells, other than international ethical guidelines, existed and just like any other medical practices the research was regulated under the Medical Practitioners Law, which is the legal basis of the medical licensing system in Japan. Under this law, the doctors reserve the discretionary right to decide how their patients ought to be treated, and are allowed to use drugs and devices not yet approved by the government. The condition for conducting clinical studies of regenerative medicine was only that both the patient and their cells had to remain under a doctor's control throughout the procedure. For this reason, the cells had to be cultured at a hospital. In other words, the collaboration for cell sheet therapy could not have taken place if the surgeon had been unable to offer the space for culturing the cells.

Hospital-based collaborations like this produced some clinically promising results but advances in clinical applications of adult stem cells have seldom led to commercial applications. As Okano's spin-off company represents, commercial actors existed already in the early 2000s and many of them contributed to such collaborations in one way or another. However, for them, initiating the similar research procedure would have been a different issue. In clinical trials, for instance, companies must follow the Pharmaceutical Affairs Law, regulating manufacturing of drugs and devices, as well as the instructions of the Ministry of Health and Welfare (MHW)[4] on cellular products. The instructions (MHW, 1999) stipulate that a company must demonstrate both safety and efficacy of its product to start the

---

4   The MHW was re-structured as the Ministry of Health, Labour and Welfare (MHLW) in the 2001 Central Government Reform.

phase-I clinical trial. However, as some company-based researchers complain, this requirement is not easy to meet. Firstly, efficacy may not be evident, even for the company, as pre-clinical studies only demonstrate the results from animal models and their relevance to human subjects is uncertain. Secondly, without clear criteria for product safety, the company is expected to be accountable for its product beyond its production line. Unlike in clinical research, a product must be delivered to a hospital, and the company has to demonstrate that its cellular product remains stable and safe even for this extra period of time. Furthermore, the company has to conduct the entire procedure in a strictly controlled working environment, which was not a condition necessary for clinical research at hospitals.[5] Therefore, despite their participation in the research cluster, many companies were not able to take advantage of it.

The Birth of Induced Pluripotent Stem Cells

Until 2006, the two clusters co-existed with little interactions in Japanese regenerative medicine research. One was the cluster of stem cell scientists, emphasising the biological mechanisms of cellular development, differentiation and regeneration, progressed with the government support since the beginning of the new millennium; and the other was that of biomedical engineers and medical doctors, who focused on the therapeutic use of adult somatic cells, with some success on treating patients but not on delivering products to the market. However, neither of these clusters was able to present its legitimacy in this emerging field and to represent regenerative medicine research: the former cluster failed to produce clinically useful knowledge that the government demanded, and the latter only operated in a small scale under the privileged status of licensed doctors. The distance between the two clusters appeared as though the conventional division of 'basic' and 'applied' research was at work and was large as ever. However, the situation started to change in late 2006 when Shinya Yamanaka's research group invented a novel technique to reprogram the biological characters of adult cells and created what they called iPS cells from mouse skin cells.

Yamanaka and his colleague Kazutoshi Takahashi (2006) argued that their technique had the potential to resolve ethical issues of hES cell research because their cells exhibited the identical biological properties as ES cells, but there was a question about its applicability to human cells at that time. If only applicable to non-human animals, this technique would not differ much from previous cloning techniques and would fail to confirm its clinical relevance – from the government's perspective, this could have been merely another achievement in

---

5   This policy gap between academic clinical research and industrial clinical trials existed until 2006, when the MHLW introduced its Guidelines on Clinical Research using Human Stem Cells, setting the similar standards for clinical research in hospitals (Guidelines, 2006; and also Matsuyama, 2008).

pure science. In 2007, however, Yamanaka succeeded in applying this technique to human skin cells and successfully demonstrated its potential clinical relevance (Takahashi et al., 2007). Within a couple of days of this announcement, MEXT sent its officers to Yamanaka to evaluate the implications of the technique and discuss how the Ministry could support his research further (Hishiyama, 2010). As Thomson's group in the US also reported its success in creating human iPS cells almost at the same time (Yu et al., 2007), MEXT sensed the intensity of international competition in this field and took responsibility for supporting his research, simultaneously allowing itself to claim credit for its future advancement.

Within the couple of months since Yamanaka's announcement, the government held several meetings and he was invited to explain how useful iPS cells would be for regenerative medicine and drug development. In these meetings, he suggested that forming a collaborative research network would be indispensable if Japan were to compete against research universities in the US and elsewhere (Hishiyama, 2010). MEXT adopted this vision and established the 'All-Japan' research network for iPS cell research. Central to this network were the Center for iPS Cell Research and Application (CiRA), a research institute founded at Kyoto University for and directed by Yamanaka, and MEXT's Project for Realization of Regenerative Medicine. The Project started its second term in April 2008, and Yamanaka joined the three principal figures by becoming its fourth core researcher. With these developments, the focus of this project also shifted from multipotent stem cells to iPS cells, and Shinichi Kousaka, a senior medical scientist was appointed the new project leader. Yamanaka also became the director of two other research programmes focusing on iPS cells, one with the support of MEXT and the other with that of the Cabinet Office. Here, the collaborative network of iPS cell research was established under the government's initiative. While the members belong to different universities and research centres, they were expected to share their latest findings and research resources within this network and maintain Japan's leading position in this emerging field.

In addition to the political support, Yamanaka also enjoyed great public support. The news about his creation of human iPS cells circulated widely in the Japanese mass media – that a young Japanese scientist invented a new technique, resolving one of the significant challenges in cutting-edge life science, immediately brought massive popularity (cf., Shineha et al., 2010). Compliments from well-recognised political and religious leaders, like the US President and the Pope, also helped this phenomenon. The concept that iPS cells could allow one's cells to be utilised for treating one's own disease, thereby alleviating the problem of organ shortage, was another reason for its popularity in this country. To maintain and potentially increase this public support, MEXT has frequently held public events around its programmes of regenerative medicine research since the end of 2007, and all have been very well attended. The scene of audiences taking photos of Yamanaka has been common in such events, indicating Yamanaka's 'heroic' status, representing not only Japanese regenerative medicine research but also the community of science. His popularity among the public served to re-vitalise the cluster of stem cell scientists and MEXT promised them another five years of its support, despite their persistent struggle to produce clinically useful knowledge.

During this remarkable period for the cluster of stem cell scientists, hospital-based collaborations also made some progress. Only several weeks after Yamanaka's announcement of creating human iPS cells, Sawa announced that his first myoblast-therapy patient had made a fast recovery and was de-hospitalised. Almost simultaneously, a start-up company Japan Tissue Engineering Co. Ltd. (J-TEC) completed the series of clinical trials and obtained manufacturing authorisation for its cellular-based product for the first time in Japan. Among commercial actors, this latter event was considered particularly as an important milestone for regenerative medicine in this country, as it demonstrated that culturing cells for therapeutic use was no longer confined to a laboratory space within hospitals. The scale of the political support as well as the growing public support to iPS cell research, however, did not prove advantageous to this cluster. Despite the progress made both at a hospital and in the industry, the impact of Yamanaka's success was so significant that the term 'iPS cell research' became used synonymously with regenerative medicine research in this country. This by no means suggests that Okano's research group did not receive any government support for its research – Okano also obtained a large grant for his cell sheet engineering to realise his vision of an 'organ factory' (CAO, 2009) – yet, neither Sawa nor Okano enjoyed the public support comparable to that of Yamanaka and iPS cell research.

In 2009, MEXT, being responsible for advancing iPS cell research and accountable for a substantial portion of its financial spending, published a roadmap illustrating the future trajectory of iPS cell research over then ensuing 10 years (2009). This trajectory reflected the visions that Yamanaka explicated originally in 2007 (cf., Hishiyama, 2010), and this document was produced after consultations with the key figures in the All-Japan research network for iPS cell research. It listed four research streams: two are mainly concerned about the quality of iPS cells, with the goals of improving the reprogramming technique and producing standardised cell lines; the other two focus largely on applications, with the visions of the cells to be utilised in drug discovery and as regenerative medicine. However, it was soon revealed that the timelines suggested in this roadmap were almost impossible to meet – even from the viewpoints of the members of the research network. While stem cell scientists appeared to have achieved their legitimacy in this field owing to both political and public support, there was a growing concern among them that another failure to meet the expectation can easily overturn this situation.

A major reason for this perceived impossibility was that collaboration necessary for attaining the goals set out in the roadmap proved difficult to implement. To promote the use of iPS cells for drug discovery, for example, the cells obtained from patients must be stocked at a cell bank and made available within the network. However, many researchers were reluctant to deposit their iPS cells until they publish several articles on them. Despite MEXT's political attempt to set common goals for the iPS cell research network and to turn its projects into 'big science' working toward them, the researchers had little incentive, if any, to share their valuable resources because their personal as well as project's merit was evaluated on the basis of peer-reviewed publications and possibly on the number of patents. Principal investigators, moreover, could not afford to let publication opportunities slip away, as they were responsible for the careers of their junior laboratory members. While this resource sharing problem did not totally abandon the cross-laboratory collaborations in the field, the researchers had to be careful choosing with whom they collaborate, necessarily involving a formal mode of contract, such as material transfer agreement, just as the conventional 'small' life science research. Therefore, the laboratory-oriented style of stem cell science posed a major hurdle for developing 'big-science' collaboration that Yamanaka and MEXT envisioned in establishing their All-Japan network of iPS cell researchers.

Bridging the Gap by Building a Highway

Having publicised its expected trajectory in iPS cell research in 2009, MEXT became desperate to meet its targets. Some progress were made in the studies for improving the reprogramming technique and also for standardising iPS cells, as they were projects that Yamanaka and his new research centre CiRA played the central roles. Yamanaka's public popularity, coupled with his medical background, also gave him access to some rare disease patients and allowed his group to advance drug discovery research using the cells obtained from them, though the scale of this work seem smaller than originally planned.[6] A significant delay was observed particularly in the research stream for applications of iPS cells as regenerative medicine, and only a few areas, such as retinal regeneration, are expected to start their clinical research in the coming years. To reduce this delay, MEXT and the Ministry of Health, Labour and Welfare (MHLW) launched a new programme called the Regenerative Medicine Highway in 2011.

This Highway programme was originally proposed by MEXT (2010) to overcome what it called the 'Death Valley' in regenerative medicine, which prevents the transition from basic to applied research. In this programme, the two ministries harmonise their financial and other support for selected research projects and allow them to make seamless transitions from pre-clinical to clinical studies – a change needed to hasten the development of regenerative medicine. MEXT called for proposals in four distinctive categories: short-term projects aiming to start clinical research within three years; mid- or long-term projects targeting clinical research in five to seven years; projects set to provide technical support for research initiatives, including the Project for Realization of Regenerative Medicine; and projects studying and resolving the ethical challenges

---

6   Kyoto University established the Division for iPS Cell Application Development within its hospital in 2011 to be the contact point for patients willing to donate cells for iPS cell research.

in regenerative medicine. Thus, the Highway programme is designed not only to provide policy support to independent research projects but also to establish common resources for their smooth running, and in the first selection procedure, a total of 10 projects were chosen for its funding.

Among these 10 projects, four were short-term and four were mid- and long-term. Overall, four of the 10 focus on clinical applications of iPS cells; yet retinal regeneration was the only such study selected for the short-term,[7] reflecting delayed progress in iPS cell research. The three other short-term projects aim to develop clinical applications of adult stem and somatic cells, instead of iPS cells, and all have a medical researcher at a university hospital as their principal investigator, indicating the two ministries' intention to integrate the two clusters. Furthermore, a project aiming to develop clinical applications of hES cells was also selected for the mid- and long-term projects, alongside the three others focusing on iPS cells.[8] As it was once commonly suggested that iPS cells would eliminate the need for hES cells, the inclusion of this research project within the Highway programme indicates a dramatic shift in the field of regenerative medicine research in Japan: investigators and funders alike are becoming more open to different styles of practices, so long as they are considered to be promising avenues for its advancement with some clinical relevance.

Neither Okano nor Yamanaka is part of this Highway programme. Yet, a few projects aim to combine cell sheet engineering and iPS cells, and the medical researchers leading such projects, including Sawa, may bridge the gap that for a decade existed between the two clusters in this country. This application-oriented programme also allows commercial actors to participate, though they still perform supportive roles in the projects. While it is a collection of independent research projects, the collaboration between MEXT and the MHLW in the policy domain has provided some common grounds for regenerative medicine research and seemed to have created an accommodating environment for different styles of practices.

This shift, however, does not seem to bring about the convergence of the two clusters. In a MEXT committee meeting on stem cell science and regenerative medicine research in early 2012, a committee member commented that too much attention has been paid to iPS cells – particularly to their clinical applications – and that the abovementioned Highway programme to some extent relieved the burden on stem cell scientists, allowing them to retain their original interest in

---

7   This research project is led by Masayo Takahashi at RIKEN CDB and the clinical studies are to be conducted at the neighbouring hospital, justifying its establishment about a decade ago in the Millennium Project and its visibility in regenerative medicine research since then.

8   MEXT (2009) revised the Guidelines for Derivation and Utilization of Human Embryonic Stem Cells in 2009 and clinical applications of pluripotent stem cells, including both hES cells and iPS cells, became permitted, but the main reason behind this decision was to allow those of iPS cells.

the biological mechanisms of stem cells. This comment indicates that the bridge between the two clusters is leading to their re-configuration, instead of their convergence: only the part of iPS cell research that is more compatible with the goal-oriented style of the other cluster is segregated from the mainstream stem cell science and can be merged with the cluster developed in university hospitals. Hence, this re-configuration would not only allow stem cell scientists to maintain their original style of pure science but also legitimise it by dissociating them from the policy emphasis on producing clinically useful knowledge.

Again, this was not what Yamanaka envisioned when he proposed the All-Japan iPS cell research network back in late 2007, and his dissatisfaction with the state of collaboration in regenerative medicine research in Japan prompted him to recruit established researchers from other research groups within the network and enlarged his community at CiRA. To overcome the challenges that laboratory-based stem cell science posed for turning Japanese regenerative medicine research into 'big science', he attempts to expand his research group and cover most aspects of iPS cell research at his centre. Establishing himself as a leader of iPS cell research may be an effective approach to facilitate research coordination in this field and direct it toward the goals that he envisioned and MEXT publicised, but, as suggested at the beginning of this chapter, there can be cost in 'big science' – at least, he becomes responsible for the careers of a large number of researchers, many of whom have to obtain a new post before the government funding ends. Whether he will succeed in both coordinating research activities and attaining the original goals remains uncertain.

Discussion and Conclusion

In her study of research collaboration, Maienschein describes that 'researchers collaborate for a variety of intellectual and social reasons: to get help, to combine expertise, to gain credibility, or to create a community' (1993: 182). While each of these reasons may be applicable in any instance of research collaboration, the consistent rationale for collaborations in regenerative medicine research in Japan seems to have been the quest for legitimacy. To understand this, it is important to distinguish 'legitimacy' from 'credibility'. In their ethnographic study, Latour and Woolgar (1979) argue that the circle of credit is central to research and that scientists invest their credit, obtained from various activities in research, in earning themselves the right to do more research – for instance, by obtaining research grants, buying the latest equipment and publishing journal articles. In collaboration, Maienschein (1993) also suggests, credibility may also be shared and expanded. Thus, 'credibility' in science works like one's property, which can be obtained, possessed, invested and even shared. From this point of view, the idea of credibility resembles Bourdieu's (1999) idea of 'scientific capital', which functions just like other kinds of social capital, while specific to the 'field' of science: one accumulates by living as part of the community – receiving trainings, conducting research and presenting its result allow one to be recognised as part of the community from the peers. In contrast, 'legitimacy', for Bourdieu (1999), is about the power within the community, which must be achieved by accumulating scientific capital and possibly other social ones relevant to a field of science and ought to be exercised by influencing the peers. Achieving legitimacy is important because it is about the power not only to set the rules of its community but also to define the field.

One's scientific capitals can only be valuable so long as the community follows the same rule and recognise their value (see also Albert and Kleinman, 2011). In an interdisciplinary field, like regenerative medicine research, however, the rules are not clear – researchers may adopt different rules (cf., Panofsky, 2011). Furthermore, in this Japanese context, the value of scientific capitals seemed depreciated when stem cell science became part of the Millennium Genome Projects in 2000. The strong commitment of the government and its emphasis on 'clinically useful' knowledge forced stem cell scientists to adopt new rules of the game. However, with the structure of its community remained the same, they simply followed the original rules of 'pure' science, in which scientific credibility counts the most, and pursued their research on biological mechanisms of cellular development, differentiation and regeneration, mostly based on animal models. A few years later, they were criticised for not being 'clinically relevant'. Despite their credibility accumulated during the Millennium policy initiative, they therefore failed to achieve legitimacy and set their own rules of the game. MEXT then launched the Project for Realization of Regenerative Medicine in 2003 urging them to re-structure the community, again insisting the importance of clinical usefulness. Yet again, they struggled to team up with medical doctors, who do not value their scientific capitals much, resulting in upholding of their own cluster.

In contrast to such struggle of stem cell scientists, biomedical engineers experienced little difficulties working with active surgeons. They had been developing novel techniques on less complex adult somatic cells, and some of the techniques were quite ready for clinical studies. Surgeons, interested in treating patients primarily, were willing to collaborate with them and to test such techniques. This hospital-based collaboration was only possible where patients agree to participate in the studies, and hence patient participation served as the valuable social capital for them, indicating relevance of their research as regenerative medicine. However, they were not successful enough (or maybe they were not fast enough) to achieve legitimacy and set the rules in the field: their collaborations remained confined to hospitals spaces, where the discretionary right of medical doctors is reserved.

This situation changed dramatically in 2007 when Yamanaka announced the creation of human iPS cells. The development of the reprogramming technique in 2006 allowed him to accumulate credibility within the community of stem cell science, and then by demonstrating its applicability to human cells he successfully translated this credibility into social capital relevant to the field of regenerative medicine research. Unlike hospital-based collaborations, he has not been able to acquire much social capital of patient participation through iPS cell research, but instead by publicising his visions of using the new cells for drug discovery and as regenerative medicine he managed to frame the general public as a group of potential patients, who would benefit from advances in iPS cell research, and turn their support as the evidence of its clinical relevance. As discussed in the sociology of expectations (e.g. Brown et al., 2000; Brown and Michael, 2003), he mobilised resources in the present by presenting a scenario of the future – the enthusiastic support from healthy members of the public might not have been recognised as the valuable 'capital', unless they recognised usefulness of his research and accepted that it was clinical rather than basic (cf., Shineha et al., 2010).

MEXT attempted to affirm Yamanaka's legitimacy and make his visions as the basis of the new rules in this field by establishing the All-Japan network for iPS cell research. Yet, its attempt failed: the tension arisen within the network left the visions 'unrealistic' and hence its future value left unverified. The Ministry reacted to this by launching another programme with the MHLW. Their goal-oriented Highway programme, as discussed in the studies of innovation policy (e.g. Gibbons et al., 1994), enrolled diverse actors, including not only the members of the stem cell science cluster but also those of the other cluster, who have accumulated capitals of patient participation over the years. To some extent, MEXT managed to bridge the gap between the two clusters. Yet, some stem cell scientists considered this programme as a long-awaited opportunity to re-establish their own field where credibility is intertwined closely with legitimacy, that is, the ideal world of 'pure' science (cf., Bourdieu, 1999). Yamanaka, rather than participating in this programme and becoming part of the re-configured cluster, upholds his original visions of iPS cell research and tries to protect his legitimacy by expanding his own research centre.

According to Gieryn (1983), scientists often demonstrate their legitimacy by drawing the boundary against 'non-science' and by presenting themselves as the producers of 'valuable' knowledge. In other words, they maintain the value of credibility in science by purifying the community (Bourdieu, 1999). However, as this study of regenerative medicine research in Japan shows, the value of life science research is increasingly tied to its 'clinical relevance', and patient participation is becoming a major resource for one's legitimacy. The boundaries of the clusters in this field therefore have been drawn and re-drawn to integrate the figures of patients as its main capitals. The integration of patient figures and hence the demonstration of clinical relevance, however, are more compatible with some styles of practice than others. Thus, biomedical engineers and surgeons have been able to maintain their style at the same time as they accumulate their capitals, while stem cell scientists insisting on their own style struggled to achieve legitimacy. Despite their dramatic revival since late 2007, some stem cell scientists have been keen to re-draw a boundary again between 'basic' and 'applied' research so as to go back to where they started in 2000.

This study also demonstrates that a field of science is being shaped not only by the researchers' attempt to draw its boundaries but also by the government's attempts to justify their policy decisions. This government's influence to some extent confirms mutual reliance between science and policy (e.g. Jasanoff, 1990; Shackley and Wynne, 1995), but it seems important for the government to commit the right kind of a cluster, or otherwise it needs to make the one it already committed right because researchers tend to form different clusters. This rightness again has to be defined by the rules of the game in the field. The Japanese government's commitment with stem cell science in early 2000s could have proved successful if this field was simply of 'pure' science: the researchers made significant advancement and obtained scientific credibility since the beginning of the new millennium. However, the emphasised importance of 'clinical relevance' posed it a significant challenge. Yamanaka's creation of human iPS cells provided the government an opportunity to re-configure the cluster and justify its commitment after its unsuccessful attempts of the Millennium Genome Projects and the Project for Realization of Regenerative Medicine.

However, the initiatives on iPS cell research also turned out to be not as successful as expected because of the persistent tension within the established research network. In his study of molecular biologists, Hackett (2005) argues that such tension is critical part of 'cooperative competition' in life science. Each research group in the network wanted to make breakthroughs and obtain credibility in the field, but staying in the cluster was a strategic decision for it to have access to newly created iPS cells and enjoy the substantial research support. Before it discloses its findings and shares the data and materials produced in its research, however, the group needs to make sure that it takes full advantage of them and is better positioned in setting the rules in the field than its cooperating competitors. While Chompalov and his colleagues argue that those 'who produces an innovative [style of practice] could well be making the collaboration's task more difficult' (2002: 760), therefore, researchers in an emerging field like this have strong motivation to develop an innovative style and set the rules for the field. This kind of tension might have been resolved, just like the healthy tension within a single laboratory, if the network had a clear 'leader' to take control over activities of its members.

This policy failure provided the background for Yamanaka's gradual shift away from the 'participatory' national network to the formal hierarchy at his research centre CiRA. As a director of the centre, Yamanaka is able to set rules and coordinate the work of its members toward the shared goals, reflecting his own visions. This can also be seen as a case of 'mezzo' science emerged from the bigger one (cf., Vermeulen et al., 2010). This kind of intra-organisational collaboration can be advantageous in several ways: its formal structure can introduce the division of labour among the researchers, which 'ensures a more effective use of their talents' (Katz and Martin, 1997: 14); their physical proximity can also allow them to share their skills and tacit knowledge, which may not be conveyed through published journal articles (Katz and Martin, 1997), and finally sharing of limited time and space of research facilities, just as the case of an accelerator laboratories (Champalov et al., 2002), would prompt them to have more communications. As a director of the centre, Yamanaka is also able to adopt a different set of criteria for assessing the contribution of each member from that agreed within the cluster of regenerative medicine research. Just as MEXT and the MHLW designed in their programme, building technical and ethical resources available for its member researchers is considered to be critical for advancing this field further and Yamanaka seems keen to develop such non-scientific expertise within his research centre too.

Coordinating research activities of researchers can be a daunting task, but as Hackett (2005) suggest, a leader does not have to be good at everything but only needs to be good at articulation work, allowing its members to be part of the project with confidence in their future. The coming years will be a testament to coordination skills of Yamanaka, who have already shown his scientific excellence.

Thus, the 2012 JSRM public lecture was not only a showcase of the state-of-the-art research in this field but also that of the research clusters of which it consisted. Yamanaka engaged Takuro Tatsumi representing healthy members of the public, explained the values of his iPS cell research to the audiences and left the room. Having achieved the heroic status among the public, he had other businesses to do to maintain his legitimacy and to keep his research going. Left in the room were the two other academic speakers, Okano and Sawa. The biomedical engineer talked about his research accomplishments, which might be of interest to both academic researchers and commercial actors sitting in the room, who could be his future collaborators; their technical complication, however, discouraged most public audience to engage with his research directly. In contrast, the surgeon managed not only to demonstrate his past engagement with actual patients but also to build the link between the biomedical engineer and the public audience, serving as a 'host' for both. All the speakers tried to demonstrate their legitimacy in this underdetermined field of regenerative medicine research, but they did so in different ways reflecting their views on what is (and ought to be) valued in the field. Needless to say, no other stem cell scientist than Yamanaka spoke in this lecture, as he would have insisted that legitimacy could only be achieved by convincing fellow scientists and earning credibility from them, rather than engaging with the public audience.

References

11th Congress of JSRM 2012. *Challenge for Innovation*, 11th Congress of the Japanese Society for Regenerative Medicine, http://www2.convention. co.jp/11jsrm, retrieved 18 April 2013.

Albert, M. and Kleinman, D.L. 2011. Bringing Pierre Bourdieu to science and technology studies. *Minerva*, 49(3), 263–73.

Bourdieu, P. 1999. The specificity of the scientific field and the social conditions of the progress of reason. In: M. Biagioli (ed.) *the Science Studies Reader*. London: Routledge, 31–50.

Brown, N., Rappart, B. and Webster, A. 2000. *Contested Futures: A Sociology of Prospective Techno-Science*. Farnham: Ashgate.

Brown, N. and Michael, M. 2003. A sociology of expectations: Retrospecting prospects and prospecting retrospects. *Technology Analysis and Strategic Management*, 15(1), 3–18.

Cabinet Office 1995. *Science and Technology Basic Law*.

Cabinet Office 1996. *Science and Technology Basic Plan (1996–2000)*.

Cabinet Office 2001. *Science and Technology Basic Plan (2001–2005)*.

Cabinet Office 2009. *Saisentan Kenkyu Kaihatsu Shien Puroguramu no Kasoku, Kyoka ni kansuru Taishoukadai oyobi Haibungaku*, http://www8.cao.go.jp/cstp/output/iken100716.pdf, retrieved 18 April 2013.

Cambrosio, A., Keating, P., Schlich, T. and Weisz, G. 2006. regulatory objectivity and the generation and management of evidence in medicine. *Social Science and Medicine*, 63(1), 189–99.

Champalov, I., Genuth, J. and Shrum, W. 2002. The organization of scientific collaborations. *Research Policy*, 31(5) 749–67.

Fujimura, J.H. and Chou, D.Y. 1994. Dissent in science: Styles of scientific practice and controversy over the cause of AIDS. *Social Science and Medicine*, 38(8), 1017–36.

Galison, P. 1992. Introduction: The many faces of big science. In: P. Galison and B. Hevley (eds) *Big Science: The Growth of Large-Scale Research*. Stanford, CA: Stanford University Press, 1–17.

Galison, P. and Havley, B. 1992. *Big Science: The Growth of Large-Scale Research*. Stanford, CA: Stanford University Press.

Gibbons, M., Limoges, C., Nowotny, H., Schwartzman, S., Scott, P. and Trow, M. 1994. *The New Production of Knowledge: The Dynamics of Science and Research in Contemporary Society*. London: Sage Publications Ltd.

Gieryn, T.F. 1983. Boundary work and the demarcation of science from non-science: Strains and interests in professional ideologies of scientists. *American Sociological Review*, 48(6), 781–95.

Gottweis, H., Salter, B. and Waldby, C. 2009. *The Global Politics of Human Embryonic Stem Cell Science: Regenerative Medicine in Transition*. Basingstoke: Palgrave Macmillan.

Hackett, E.J. 2005. Essential tensions: Identity, control, and risk in research. *Social Studies of Science*, 35(5), 787–826.

Hayashi, F. and Prescott, E.C. 2002. The 1990s in Japan: A lost decade. *Review of Economic Dynamics*, 5(1), 415–31.

Hishiyama, Y. 2010. *Raifu Saiensu Seisaku no Genzai*. Tokyo: Keiso Shobo.

Ministry of Health and Welfare 1999. *The MHW Instructions No. 906 on the Quality and Safety Assurance of Medical Devices and Drugs using Cells and Tissues*, Pharmaceuticals and Medical Devices Agency, http://www.pmda.go.jp/operations/shonin/info/report/saibousosikisinsei/file/906goutuuti.pdf, retrieved 18 April 2013.

Jasanoff, S. 1990. *The Fifth Branch: Science Advisers As Policymakers.* Cambridge, MA: Harvard University Press.

Kantei 1999. *Mireniamu Purojekuto ni tsuite,* Prime Minister of Japan and His Cabinet, http://www.kantei.go.jp/jp/mille/991222millpro.pdf, retrieved 18 April 2013.

Kantei 2003. *Mireniamu Genomu Purojekuto: Purojekuto Zenhan no Chukan Hyouka – Hyouka Houkokusyo,* Prime Minister of Japan and His Cabinet, http://www.kantei.go.jp/jp/mille/genomu/zenhan/report.pdf, retrieved 18 April 2013.

Kantei 2006. *Mireniamu Genomu Purojekuto – Saisyu Hyouka Houkokusyo,* Prime Minister of Japan and His Cabinet, http://www.kantei.go.jp/jp/mille/genomu/report/17report.pdf, retrieved 18 April 2013.

Katz, J. and Martin, B. 1997. What is research collaboration. *Research Policy,* 26(1), 1–18.

Kelves, J.D. 1995. *The Physicists: The History of a Scientific Community in Modern America.* Cambridge, MA: Harvard University Press.

Latour, B. and Woolgar, S. 1979. *Laboratory Life: The Construction of Scientific Facts.* Princeton, NJ: Princeton University Press.

Lock, M. 2002. *Twice Dead: Organ Transplants and the Reinvention of Death.* Berkeley, LA: University of California Press.

Maienschein, J. 1993. Why collaborate? *Journal of the History of Biology,* 26(2), 167–83.

Matsuyama, A. 2008. An overview of 'the guideline for clinical research using human stem cells'. *Nippon Rinsho,* 66(5), 843–9.

Ministry of Education, Culture, Sports, Science and Technology 2001. *Guidelines for Derivation and Utilization of Human Embryonic Stem Cells.*

Ministry of Education, Culture, Sports, Science and Technology 2009. *iPS Saibou Kenkyu Roodomappu,* http://www.mext.go.jp/b_menu/houdou/21/06/__icsFiles/afieldfile/2009/07/15/1279621_1_1.pdf, retrieved 18 April 2013.

Ministry of Education, Culture, Sports, Science and Technology 2010. *Heisei 23 nen-do ni muketa Kansaibou Saisei Igaku kankei no Torikumi ni tsuite,* http://www.lifescience.mext.go.jp/files/pdf/n613_01.pdf, retrieved 18 April 2013.

Ministry of Health, Labour and Welfare 2006. *Guidelines on Clinical Research Using Human Stem Cells.*

Morrison, M. 2012. Promissory futures and possible pasts: The dynamics of contemporary expectations in regenerative medicine. *BioSocieties,* 7(1), 3–22.

Nakatsuji, N. 2007. Irrational Japanese regulations hinder human embryonic stem cell research. *Nature Reports Stem Cells,* 9 August 2007, http://www.nature.com/stemcells/2007/0708/070809/full/stemcells.2007.66.html, retrieved 18 April 2013.

Okano, T., Yamada, N., Okuhara, M., Sakai, H. and Sakurai, Y. 1995. Mechanism of cell detachment from temperature-modulated, hydrophilic-hydrophobic polymer surfaces. *Biomaterials,* 16(4), 297–303.

Panofsky, A.L. 2011. Field analysis and interdisciplinary science: Scientific capital exchange in behavior genetics. *Minerva*, 49(3), 295–316.

Penders, B., Horstman, K. and Vos, R. 2008. Walking the line between lab and computation: The 'moist' zone. *BioScience*, 57(8), 747–55.

Rubin, B.P. 2008. 'Therapeutic promise' in the discourse of human embryonic stem cell research. *Science as Culture*, 17(1), 13–27.

Shackley, S. and Wynne, B. 1995. Global climate change: The mutual construction of an emerging science-policy domain. *Science and Public Policy*, 22(4), 218–30.

Shineha, R., Kawakami, M., Kawakami, K., Nagata, M., Tada, T. and Kato, K. 2010. Familiarity and prudence of the Japanese public with research into induced pluripotent stem cells, and their desire for its proper regulation. *Stem Cell Reviews and Reports*, 6(1), 1–7.

Stephens, N., Atkinson, P. and Glasner, P. 2008. The UK Stem Cell Bank: Securing the past, validating the present, protecting the future. *Science as Culture*, 17(1), 43–56.

Takahashi, K., Tanabe, K., Ohnuki, M., Narita, M., Ichisaka, T., Tomoda, K. and Yamanaka, S. 2007. Induction of pluripotent stem cells from adult human fibroblasts by defined factors. *Cell*, 131, 861–72.

Takahashi, K. and Yamanaka, S. 2006. Induction of pluripotent stem cells from mouse embryonic and adult fibroblast cultures by defined factors. *Cell*, 126, 663–76.

Vermeulen, N., Parker, J.N. and Penders, B. 2010. Big, small or mezzo? Lessons from science studies for the ongoing debate about 'big' versus 'little' research projects. *EMBO Reports*, 11(6), 420–23.

Weinberg, A.M. 1961. Impact of large-scale science on the United States. *Science*, 134, 161–4.

Yu, J., Vodyanik, M.A., Smuga-Otto, K., Antosiewicz-Bourget, J., Frane, J.S., Tian, S., Nie, J., Jonsdottir, G.A., Ruotti, V., Stewart, R., Slukvin, I.I. and Thomson, J.A. 2007. Induced pluripotent stem cell lines derived from human somatic cells. *Science*, 318, 1917–20.

Chapter 9

Boundary-Spanning Engagements on a Neonatal Ward: Reflections on a Collaborative Entanglement between Clinicians and a Researcher

Jessica Mesman

Introduction

This chapter describes the collaborative effort of introducing the method of video reflexivity on a neonatal intensive care unit (NICU) in the Netherlands. As a specialised facility for the care and treatment of newborns the NICU admits babies when their condition requires close attention and careful monitoring, due to, for example, prematurity or life-threatening complications at birth. This tertiary care unit provides the most advanced level of care. If for more than 20 years critical care units such as emergency departments and ICUs have served as empirical contexts of my research,[1] the NICU, as a high-density zone of uncertainty, vulnerability and technology, has fascinated me as a scholar in particular. Over the years my presence on this ward has changed from doing classical ethnographic research to being an active member of one of its project groups, the video team.

To discuss my collaboration with the clinicians of the neonatology ward, it is first relevant to take a closer look at different aspects of collaboration as discussed in the literature.[2] Studies of collaboration refer to a diverse set of relevant characteristics, such as interrelationships and interaction, exposure and exchange, shared or diverse interest, diversity and complementarity of expertise, parity regarding responsibility and outcome, enhancement of quality and/or quantity, autonomy of partners and ownership, the importance of trust and the potential for tensions.[3] Whether these characteristics are present and in

---

1   Topics of analysis were, for example, uncertainty, ethical concerns, patient safety, spatial analysis, reflections on method, and collaboration among care providers. For studies on collaborative practices in critical care, see Mesman (2007; 2008; 2010; 2012b).

2   The notion 'clinicians' refers to health care practitioners and as such involves doctors as well as nurses.

3   See for example Amabile et al. (2001), Clark et al. (1996), Fortun and Cherkasy (1998), Katz and Martin (1997), and Morris and Hebden (2008).

what form depends on the kind of collaboration. For example, a project based on 'horizontal collaboration', that is among peers (Paules, Woodside and Ziegler, 2010), has another distribution of responsibility and ownership than one based on a more hierarchical relationship. Furthermore, it also makes a difference whether participants either share the same objective and work together towards a common product (Maienschein, 1993) or 'cooperate', that is work together without a shared objective (Shrum, Genuth and Chompalov, 2007).

In order to organise my argument in this chapter I will first discuss motives for collaboration and how they can be different and similar at the same time. Next I will describe the constitution of the core elements of the collaborative framework involved that is the content and the key players. This will also show the importance of actors who are not always directly involved. After this description of the selection process of the topic and the diversity of the actors, my argument in the fifth section shifts towards the effects of the outcome of the collaborative project on the collaboration process itself, revealing not only the entanglement of health care practice, research practice and collaborative practice, but also that the output is not always on the level of the selected topic. Collaboration, as the sixth section will discuss, turns out to be self-replicating because it generates more collaboration. In the final section I address collaboration as a 'doing', as something that intervenes. As such collaboration requires attention not only on the level of its content, but also as organisational form of work. Before discussing these various aspects of collaboration, however, I will first present the context in which my collaboration with the neonatology ward originated.

The NICU as a Context of Care, Competencies and a Camera

NICUs are characterised by high technology, high-intensity and high-reliability. This so-called 'high-3 work environment' (Owen, Wackers and Béguin, 2009) exemplifies very well the complexity of medical practices and the prominent role of technologies. Notwithstanding the presence of advanced technology and highly trained personnel, NICU staff is well aware that their work is a form of 'tightrope walking'. Many of their medical interventions come with the potential of turning into tricky problems because a range of technological advances in medicine have made it possible to treat ever-smaller patients. More and more NICU patients have a birth weight of around 500 grams and are born just after 25 weeks of gestational age. This vulnerability turns NICU work into 'risky business' that requires a careful management of the delicate balance between providing 'safe care' and providing 'effective treatment'. Finding and maintaining this balance positions patient safety in the foreground of attention of NICU staff.

For some years now patient safety has had my full attention. Whereas in health care the focus of patient safety research is on the absence of safety, that is (potential) errors and mistakes, I study the presence of safety instead. As argued elsewhere, improvement of patient safety benefits not only from the absence of risks and mistakes but also from a thorough understanding of the presence of safety (Mesman, 2012). After all, if complex practices are imperfect by nature, it is not farfetched to expect incidents to occur. This made me wonder why things do not go wrong more often. Why do we see not more errors and incidents on the NICU? How do clinicians on the NICU manage to maintain an adequate level of safety *despite* the complexity of their tasks? To work with fallible technologies and sometimes unrealistic rules or incompatible procedures while at the same time providing safe care is an accomplishment that warrants not only more appreciation, but also investigation. Apart from the intended formal measures such as built-in alarm systems, the double check of medication and a strict protocolised way of working, patient safety also involves an unarticulated – and perhaps even unplanned yet effective – set of actions and initiatives. If we are to understand the vigour and success of NICU practices, we have to explicate these non-intentionally built-in processes and structures as well as the contextual contingencies, which contribute to the constitution of patient safety. Understanding the full spectrum of ingredients of safety, then, requires an explication of the 'hidden' competencies of clinicians and their informal resources.

Identifying already existing – but often overlooked or forgotten – competencies and resources can be considered an act of 'exnovation'. Exnovation foregrounds the implicit and hidden aspects of practices (Iedema, Mesman and Carroll, 2013; Mesman, 2012; de Wilde, 2000). With its focus on ways of doing and reasoning that have gone out of sight, it acknowledges that also the mundane is crucial in the accomplishment of – in this case – reliable and safe care practices. This invisible work is of utmost importance in maintaining an adequate level of safety.[4] Unlike innovation, exnovation does not intend to bring new elements into some practice but aims to explicate and use the *already* available resources.

Moving from my research focus (doing safety) to the notion of exnovation, leads me to my final step in explaining the relationship between patient safety and collaboration: the method. What method is needed to identify 'the missing masses' of safety?[5] Let me first summarise my argument. It is my claim that the preservation of an adequate level of safety requires 'more' than well-trained clinicians, high technology and protocols. This begs the question: what is this 'more'? To exnovate these existing resources we have to focus on the ordinary, the usual, and the regular aspects of practice. Since clinicians hardly discuss those aspects of their work that go well and are safe, standard ethnography will not serve us as the most adequate route. To exnovate the hidden resources of strength in the NICU practice, it has no use to embark on a trajectory that teaches me to see the practice 'through the eyes of the insiders', because they themselves have ceased to

---

4   For more on 'invisible work' see Star (1991).

5   The idea of the 'missing masses' of safety is inspired on the article of Bruno Latour 'Where are the missing masses? The sociology of a few mundane artifacts' (1992) in which he argues that the missing masses of morality and law that control human behaviour can be found in technology.

see these resources. Such a 'practical blindness', however, does not imply that the NICU clinicians have become 'useless' in this respect. On the contrary, employing these resources implies they have access to it. As such, clinicians can act as a passageway to the 'more' that is assumed to be present. But this requires them to be able to identify their own hidden strengths. In other words, I need them and I need a method that dissolves their 'practical blindness'.

A route that facilitates exnovation is the method of 'video-reflexivity' (Iedema, Mesman and Carroll, 2013).[6] The main principle of this method is that clinicians view video footage of their own everyday work. This re-presentation of their daily routines creates a distance that enables them to see things they have forgotten or remained opaque, in new ways (Iedema et al., 2006; Carroll, 2009; Carroll, Iedema and Kerridge, 2008). Viewing and discussing video footage together generates new ways of seeing their own daily routines. By watching video fragments that display interactions at the micro-level and discussing these processes of 'health-care-in-action' that they normally take as given, clinicians can now identify their strengths (and flaws). This form of 'video-reflexive ethnography' (Carroll, Iedema and Kerridge, 2008) requires not only familiarity with the goings-on of this ward, but also knowledge of the socio-historical context of the presented video fragments (for example the unanticipated side effects of protocols). Also required is insider's knowledge of the specificities of the context's meso-level (for example organisational and financial facilitators and barriers) and macro-level (for example the organisational structure of hospital, professional values, insurances, health care system). In other words, I need them to help me open up their practice. Likewise, they need me to open up theirs. To describe this position, Iedema and Carroll (2011) have coined the concept of 'clinalyst', which is shorthand for 'outsider-analyst-catalyst' (176). A clinalyst generates insider's knowledge by asking outsider's questions.

In general the method of video-reflexivity includes several cycles of data collection and analysis. The first one involves data collection by indicating and filming relevant situations. What is considered as a relevant topic is decided, for example in the project on the neonatology ward, by the members of the video team which consists of six nurses, a physician's assistant and myself. Yet, it is agreed that all clinicians on the neonatology ward can suggest topics to be filmed. For the NICU staff situations become relevant when they are essential to infection prevention, such as proceedings related to intravenous systems. The video-recordings of these situations are analysed and edited on the basis of their usefulness for the reflexivity meeting, resulting in the selection of short, representative clips. Again, it is up to the members of the video team to select the footage that will be presented during the

---

6   This methodology was developed in the course of the HELiCS project (Iedema and Merrick, 2008) aiming to enable clinicians to improve their own communication practices. Observing and discussing their *own* handover practices on the basis of video footage of local handover situations enabled the clinicians to evaluate and redesign if necessary their handover practice.

reflexivity meetings. This selection is based on several criteria such as level of detail, clear visibility, routine or exceptional case, diversity of task execution, to name a few. Then the selected footage is replayed to their colleagues during video-reflexivity meetings in which they discuss these visualisations of their own daily practices. A compilation of the proposed suggestions for improvement is evaluated and this will act as a point of departure for quality and safety improvements. But every stage of collecting (empirical, montage and social) and analysis (recordings, footage, notes) has implications for the form and intensity of the collaboration involved.

My collaboration with the neonatology ward started many years ago. After being introduced to the method of video reflexivity by Rick Iedema and Katherine Carroll,[7] I started to film the doctors and nurses on the Dutch NICU that I studied as part of my research on patient safety. I selected the footage, organised and chaired the reflexivity meetings and taped their discussions, thus making visible the unintended and unplanned patterns of backstage processes of 'doing safety', which subsequently the clinicians could explicitly articulate. Yet, their discussions proved not only relevant for my research project. They also provided NICU staff an opportunity to improve their practice. In this way I had something to offer as well: a tool to improve patient safety on a tailor-made basis. Due to other obligations (for example teaching) I could not always be present on the ward. During these weeks the reflexivity meetings had to be cancelled because I could not prepare and organise them. The reflexivity meetings were clearly dependent on my time and presence on the NICU. To make them independent of my presence and involvement, the method had to become theirs. A year later I was in the middle of translating the reflexivity method together with a team of clinicians into a structural part of their practice. Today the reflexivity meetings on the NICU take place independently of my presence on the ward, a result that required a collaborative effort and quite some patience.

In the remainder of this chapter I will reflect on this collaborative project, in which collaboration can be found on every level and in multiple forms, especially as object of reflection and analysis. This pertains to analysis of the collaborative activities as observed and discussed by those present during the reflexivity meetings, as well as my own analysis of the collaborative activities captured by the camera. Furthermore, as part of my research project I also analysed the actors' collaborative knowledge production during reflexive meetings while they discuss the footage in order to exnovate the 'missing masses' that constitute a safe practice. Finally, there is reflection on our collaboration in this chapter. In this respect I will not discuss results of the exnovation of the 'missing masses' itself. Rather, I will focus on different aspects of the collaborative process in which the reflexive meeting turned from 'just' a 'research instrument' into 'a structural part of the ward's improvement practices'. In the next section I will first focus on the motives that buttressed our collaboration.

---

7   I participated in their video-reflexivity project about handovers on an emergency ward in New South Wales, Australia.

Pluralism as a Strategic Resource[8]

There are as many different reasons for collaboration as there are forms of collaboration. In the literature, different social and intellectual motives are described for groups or individuals to work together.[9] For example, there may be a need for a specific kind of expertise or simply just 'more hands'. In these cases we encounter notions like 'leverage', 'combining' and 'capitalizing' (Lasker, Weiss and Miller, 2001: 180). Other reasons might relate to an increase in output in terms of efficiency, creativity or the reduction of costs (ibid.: 184; Parker, Vermeulen and Penders, 2010), or to access to data or an increase of acceptability and credibility of the project. Also the creation of a (disciplinary) community, a (personal) network or the visibility of the project is considered as an important motive for collaborative projects. Last but not least collaboration is considered as a way to enhance the quality of work and output through capitalising on complementary strength by cross-fertilisation of intellectual ideas and transfer of knowledge and skills (for example Katz and Martin, 1997). Whatever reason, all of the above refer to the underlying principle of 'more-heads (and-hands)-are-better-than-one' (Maienschein, 1997: 167). Fortun and Cherkasky (1998) describe collaboration as something that 'draws people with different interests, perspectives and skills into a synchronised effort to accomplish something that could not be accomplished individually' (146). According to them, collaboration is all about 'diversity' in which we have to understand 'pluralism as a strategic resource' (ibid.). Others, like Lasker, Weiss and Miller (2001), stress this aspect of diversity as well. For them collaboration is about 'synergy': combining perspectives, resources and skills (ibid.: 183). This is reflected etymologically in the roots of the concept of collaboration: to collect, colour and to labour (Fortun and Cherkasky, 1998: 145). In other words, it refers to 'co-labouring'. According to Maienschein (1993), this brings in the minimal condition of 'working together toward a common product' (168) in order to be labelled as collaboration.[10]

What about us, the clinicians and me? Did we work together towards a common product? What about my motives for working together with the neonatology staff? And what was their motive for working with me? Did we actually have the same objective while working side-by-side on the video reflexivity project? What made me want to collaborate in another way with the clinicians that I had studied for so many years already? The answers to these questions vary with the level to which we wish to zoom in. First, as described in the previous section, it was my aim to gain access to 'hidden competencies' in order to understand the accomplishment

---

8   This heading is a quote from Fortun and Cherkasky (1998: 146).

9   On different motives for collaboration, see for example Cheek (2008), Katz and Martin (1997), Lasker, Weiss and Miller (2001), Maienschein (1993), Reeves et al. (2010) and Roper (2002).

10   Yet to talk about true or full collaboration requires, according to Maienschein (1993), equal partnership (compare section 4).

of adequate levels of safety in a complex work environment such as an intensive care unit for newborns. This objective is based on my academic project on the phenomena of practical knowledge whereby patient safety serves as a case study. To be more precise, I consider the video-reflexivity meeting as a 'knowledge-lab' where situations are reflected upon explicitly and as a collective activity. For my research project these meetings act as a detour for data collection because these meetings are one of the few places where safety (instead of incidents and errors) is articulated. The collaboration was thus meant to *create a corridor* to inside knowledge (Pinch, Collins and Carbone, 1996), allowing me to follow safety as an actor's category as a way to gain in-depth insight into the diversity of meanings and experiences of safety *in practice.* Secondly, patient safety is hardly a neutral issue of course, as it is about preventing harm and saving a patient's life. As such it has a normative appeal one cannot and, in my opinion, should not resist. Accordingly, gaining insight into the preservation of adequate levels of safety should not only be used for the sake of theory building, but should also have a direct or indirect practical application.[11] In other words, I collaborated with the neonatology staff because I sought to *make a difference* on the ward considering patient safety. According to Zuiderent (2005), collaboration with clinicians provides a basis for 'preventing implementation' (12). With this notion Zuiderent aims to move beyond the classical distinction between phases of design, implementation and evaluation of results. Instead of presenting an outsider's assessment report, one acts from within to make a difference. Making a difference from within is closely related to Lynch's notion of 'local-interactional spaces' (Lynch, 2009). Lynch encourages us to try to create local-interactional spaces in which we question the taken-for-granted, such as the social and the technical as distinct entities or the dominant images of practices, and tries to make the practitioners to (re)imagine their world.[12] This methodological approach is considered a form of on-going reflection that has its focus on the specific conceptualisation and framing of everyday practice (ibid.). We may consider the discussions in the meetings on the ward as a local interactional space in which I acted as a clinalyst and questioned (breaching) their dominant ways of understanding patient safety. In this way I use the video-reflexivity meetings to increase the 'safety sensibility' of clinicians and to offer alternative images of patient safety in order to improve patient safety. Thirdly, my collaboration was also motivated, in other words, by my aim *to build a platform* were clinicians are allowed to take the time to sit down and reflect on 'the general logic of their ways of working' and 'develop practice-relevant insights'

---

11   As such I also have to serve two audiences: a more theoretical one (with its academic audience of STS-scholars, medical sociologists and anthropologists and) and a more practical one (with its practice-based audience of doctors and nurses, hospital managers and policy makers).

12   The strategy of using local interactional spaces was proposed by Michael Lynch in the context of the debate about the 'market value' of STS during a workshop at the Saïd Business School at Oxford University (30 June 2004).

and develop a language for addressing these complexities in their daily routines (Iedema, Mesman and Carroll, 2013). With this more emancipatory-motivated objective I aim to contribute to the critical competence of the practitioners (Penders and Radstake, forthcoming) in order to turn them into constructive 'critical participants' (Downey, 2009) of their own practice.

The improvement of patient safety is a motive for collaboration that I shared with the neonatology staff. They too want to improve patient safety of course. They too want to make a difference: by further lowering the level of infection rates. With a patient population as fragile as theirs, infection prevention is part of every activity on the ward. Especially for premature babies an infection can have serious – even lethal – consequences. Therefore, the neonatology staff take every opportunity to minimise the risk of infection, even if in such indirect way as video reflexivity. From the very first day the video reflexivity was introduced on their ward the staff explicitly stated that infection prevention had to be the topic to begin with. The importance of infection prevention made it easy for them to select it as a focus for the project. Besides their own standard improvement trajectories, such as the hand hygiene protocol, they recognised the potential of video-reflexivity for patient safety and infection prevention in particular. To them our collaboration also acted as a corridor: to an instrument they wanted to make their own. They expressed their frustration that there were no reflexivity meetings during my absence. My input provided them with a way to acquire the knowledge needed to turn this method into a structural part of their enhancement practices. This would imply that the application of the method becomes independent of my presence on the ward as our collaboration was targeted to train them using the method of video reflexivity. Besides wanting to make a difference regarding infection rates and making the method their own, the clinicians had another motivation: they too wanted to build a platform. For them the reflexivity meetings could serve as a platform where they could discuss issues that frustrated them. In other words, the selection of the topics and the footage was a way to get things on the agenda.

Levels of Objectives

Both the clinicians and I aspired to create a corridor, build a platform and make a difference but we did not pursue this in the same way. In the literature on collaboration there is much attention for different ambitions within a collaborative project. In most cases they are discussed as potential causes of conflict.[13] In the case of the reflexivity project the clinicians and I shared the same motives to collaborate and there was no conflict. We all wanted to use the video reflexivity method in a way that it became independent of my involvement. In literature there are many references to collaborative projects in which the partners had a shared ambition

---

13   See for example Dooner, Mandzuk and Clifton, 2007; Hackett, 2005; Morris and Hebden, 2008; Paulus, Woodside and Ziegler, 2010; Roper, 2002; Shrum, Genuth and Chompalov, 2001.

and perspective, but nevertheless ended up in a conflict. A possible explanation for the smoothness of the collaboration between the clinicians and me was not only the fact that it was at their own request that the ward adopted the method. A crucial factor in this regard is the longstanding relationship between the NICU clinicians and myself after more than 20 years of ethnographic research. Over time we have built up a relationship that is based on mutual respect and familiarity with each other's work and ambitions. This, of course, raises the question: to what extend does this longstanding cooperation between the clinical team and me explain the lack of difficulty? After all, the hospitality of the ward for more than 20 years reflects the existence of a good relationship. Moreover, my long-term presence has contributed to my understanding of their (verbal and bodily) language, which is crucial for interpreting their responses to the project. It is, for example, important to sense when to stop filming during the day as to prevent overkill. But what about the position of a researcher who would be introduced as completely new and relatively unknown into a group of clinicians?[14] To reduce potential difficulties a bottom up approach is essential: the introduction of video reflexivity should be on request of the ward and with approval of the majority of the clinicians. Introducing this method as a top down decision is an invitation for problems. Having said this, a bottom up approach does not provide a guarantee for an unproblematic collaboration.

If we move to another analytical level, however, the idea of a shared objective dissolves. Then we may identify academic aspirations (inside knowledge) on the one side and practice-related objectives (appropriation of a method) on the other side. Also the political ambition related to the project is diverging now into one that is profession-related (empowerment of clinicians) and one that is related to the goings-on of the ward (form of agenda-setting in order to discuss practice issues). The shared aim to improve the practice is located at a different level as well: a more general one (patient safety) and a specific one (infection-prevention). In other words, on the level of the neonatology ward there was a common aim: that video reflexivity would evolve into a structural part of their practice. Yet, on the level of the reflexivity meetings our aims diverged. Their objective was to learn from each other with the help of video and, if needed, adjust their ways of working. For this reason their focus was on the content of the footage and the practical implications of their discussion. My objective, on the other hand, was on the content of their discussion while they discuss why things go well in order to identify their competencies. While their notes are about which actions to be taken, mine refer to the particularities of knowledge building and their sharing and

---

14   During the writing of this chapter I started to work with a video team on another ward. On this ward I am a complete stranger. So far there have been no problems, but it is still too soon to qualify this collaboration as one without conflicts. Also on this ward I follow the strategy of 'planned obsolescence', meaning a gradual withdrawal from the position of being in charge of the video reflexivity method in order to hand it over to the clinicians of this ward.

applying of know-how in the daily routines of a complex heath care practice. On this level, then, there was clearly neither a common goal, nor a common output and a common preparation or follow-up.

Weick (1997) views different ambitions merely as a temporal incongruence that in the end will dissolve when all ambitions converge into one.[15] Such a linear perspective seems to assume that convergence is an inherent characteristic of collaboration. In the video reflexivity project, however, motives for collaboration were diverse and they will always be so given that some of them are linked rather disparately while others overlap. Our ambitions will never evolve into one common goal that rules out differences. Moreover, as described above, the presence or absence of a common goal also depends on the level on which one wishes to zoom in. On a more general plane the different actors may have a shared objective, while on a more detailed level their objectives may differ in so many ways. Despite these differences, in the case at hand there have been no conflicts within the video team so far. A possible explanation might precisely be the presence of different levels of objectives: we shared some of them while others we did not share. Levels of objectives might create just enough suppleness to prevent tension from building, while also providing options for switching whenever needed.[16]

In general, however, adopting this reflexive instrument involves more than good intentions. It also needs room to position itself in the texture of the practice. To create this room, as I discuss in the next section, a great deal of fine-tuning and commitment is required.

Building the Collaborative Texture

The ambition is to turn the video reflexivity method into a structural part of the organisation of the neonatology practice. This requires the meetings to transform from 'an occasional happening' into 'the normal Monday meeting'. It has to become just as normal as the daily rounds or the time schedule of the different shifts. This proved no easy task because the existing practice was already overloaded with an array of tasks that had to be performed during particular moments of the day (for example observation of the patients by the nurses every two hours or the examination of the babies by the doctors before the daily round, or the daily round by doctors and nurses before noon) in specific places (for example at the bedside, in the meeting room). In other words, adopting the method means opening up the socio-geographical structure of the ward. This, however, involves a boundary-spanning engagement that goes beyond the simple notion of a collaborative act

---

15   Karl Weick's model of 'means convergence' as discussed by Dooner, Mandzuk and Clifton (2008) is a good example of this idea of linearity. This framework describes four developmental stages of collaborative practices: diverse ends, common means, common ends and diverse means.

16   One can compare it to a family house with different rooms and floors.

between a researcher and a hospital ward. A closer look reveals that in order to create the necessary socio-geographical space for the reflexivity method requires multiple collaborations and they differ substantially in nature. Hackett (2005) stresses that collaboration itself should be viewed as a socio-geographical practice that changes over time. Moreover, during the project the collaboration expanded much like a stone thrown into the pond: more and more groups got involved. In this section I will discuss the thematic focus of the project, the extent and heterogeneity of the collaborative process by describing the different steps that in this particular case were taken to implement the video reflexivity method on the ward.

Redefining the Thematic Focus of Collaboration

My successful meeting with one of the managing directors of the hospital, as described in the previous section, resulted in a contractual agreement between the hospital and the university. The next step to be taken was to meet with the management team of the neonatology ward in order to discuss with them the possibility of adopting the video reflexivity method. During a meeting with members of the management team – the head-nurse, one of the neonatologists, and one of the nurse unit managers – it was immediately clear that they wanted to give it a go. Their enthusiastic response was based on a shared frustration about the fact that during my absence on the ward video reflexivity meetings were not possible. This was due to the fact that up until then it was just me who did all the filming, imported them on my pc, selected and edited the footage, organised and chaired the meetings. For them the question whether or not video reflexivity should become a structural part of the ward was not an issue at all. Everyone in the room saw it as an excellent opportunity. But we still had to decide on the content of the collaboration. To prevent 'just filming anything that moves', a clear focus was required. At the same time, the video material also had to be of interest to both parties. Considering my research project on patient safety and their vulnerable patient population it was agreed that infection prevention would serve as the overall focus with special attention for those moments and activities that are prone to 'line infections'.[17] Therefore clinicians' work should be performed with maximal cleanliness. Notwithstanding their efforts, infections are like a

---

17   Very ill or premature newborns lack the strength to feed themselves. Therefore, a small polyurethane tube is inserted into the baby's bloodstream. This catheter provides access to the baby's body to administer medication and parental nutrition. Central catheters are used when it is expected that the baby needs intravenous infusions for an extended period of time. In this way, they can avoid the stress and discomfort of repeated needle sticks because these central catheter's lines can stay in as long as three weeks. Unfortunately, the deployment of this technique is not without risk. Intravenous access can cause infections, the so-called catheter-related bloodstream infections (CRBSIs). Vascular infections make up a huge part of the hospital-acquired infections and contribute substantially to hospital morbidity and mortality rates.

'permanent resident' on the NICU.[18] Persevering in their ambitions, the NICU staff uses every opportunity to improve their practice and lower the infection rates. The video reflexivity project was one of those opportunities. It was decided to pay attention to two procedures in particular because they involve an obvious potential risk regarding line infection: the insertion of a central venous catheter and the renewal of intravenous systems.[19] Of course, it was stressed, other issues related to infection prevention would also fall within the scope of the project.

With the approval of the project and selecting a focus, for me the first meeting was an instant success. The main challenge, however, was to make myself superfluous, because others had to take over the project. Furthermore, clinicians' willingness to collaborate and take the video project seriously was *the* critical factor in the project's success. This required a collaborative relationship with the clinicians on the ward.

The Key Players

To be able to use the method independently of my presence on the ward, a video team had to be established. It was decided to involve those nurses who were already familiar with filming due to a project related to videoing parent–child interaction. Moreover, considering our focus, the nurses who participated in the working group on infection prevention were regarded as a logical choice. Aside from nurses, a medical staff member was also supposed to join the team. It was decided that the neonatologist in charge of infection prevention who also attended this first meeting would be the one. The two physician assistants (PA) on the ward would be invited to join as well.[20] Like the residents, PAs are present on the NICU all day and do much of the work. Unlike residents, PAs don't leave the ward after just a few months, but belong to the ward.

Furthermore, the method of video-reflexivity required not only the approval and commitment of the management of the ward, but also – and even more so

---

18   Estimations present figures of around 50,000 to 100,000 bloodstream infections per year in the United States alone. Ninety per cent of these infections are related to central venous catheters (Sheretz et al., 2000). To prevent CRBSI, several strategies have been developed, ranging from finding the best insertion site, skin preparation with chlorhexidine, maintaining proper nurse staffing levels and the use of catheters with anti-infective coatings or antibiotic impregnated catheters to the use of maximal barrier precautions (MBP). The optimal safety strategy is to use all of these strategies (Rubinson and Diette, 2004; Rizzo, 2005). Whatever the strategy, the various preventative actions all aim to keep the germs out by working with sterile instruments in a sterile environment.

19   This is a medical procedure that is done under sterile conditions by a doctor who is assisted by a nurse. Also the renewal of the closed intravenous system every 72 hours by the nurses would be at the centre of attention. In order to renew this device, the so-called 'Octopus', the closed system has to be opened, and this creates a moment of potential infection.

20   Although not fully trained as a medical doctor, physician assistants are allowed, to a limited extent, to execute medical procedures, but only under supervision of a physician.

– of the clinicians on the floor.[21] After all, their involvement is needed on every level: they have to allow being filmed in action and they need to reflect on the footage that is presented to them during the reflexivity meetings. This is why having them on my side was more than important: it was crucial. For this reason I started with a contextual exploration for two weeks.[22] During this time I was on the ward during different shifts in order to inform the NICU staff about the purpose and process of being filmed. Additionally, I explained to them their own role and their rights. For example, they had the right not to participate or to refuse being filmed.[23] Participation and being filmed were voluntary, and anyone could decline to be filmed at any time. In close collaboration with the hospital's legal advisor I also prepared a document which stated that none of the video material would be shown to people not involved in the project or used for individual assessment. This proviso is an integral part of standard ethics approvals, and it was particularly important to emphasise its relevance given the NICU context, with its demanding and complex work routines.

This preparatory stage hardly involved a one-way flow of information. As much as I informed the clinicians about the project, they provided advice to me about what and when to film regarding infection prevention. They came up with a host of topics, such as hand hygiene, use of personal protective equipment, but also the 'spaghetti' of lines behind the incubator that complicated their work. Based on their suggestions I made a topic list and, where possible, I added the timeslots in which these situations occurred or particular procedures were likely to be performed. In this way I sought to create a platform for collaboration – for their support, advice and involvement.

Different kinds of 'technologies of collaboration' (Hackett, 2005) are required to maintain the texture in which the key players work together. For example, an infrastructure of communication had to be established because the outcomes of the reflexivity meetings had to be communicated to the wider community of clinicians. We developed two distinct lines of communication: one for the doctors (mailing group) and one for the nurses (their weekly meetings). In addition, we needed to organise communication within the video team since most of its members, and

---

21   An application was sent to the ethical committee of the hospital to ask for their approval. However, the members of the committee decided that this project did not require their approval because it did not involve any invasive interaction with patients. Nevertheless, with the help of the hospital's legal department, I did develop and use an informed consent form for the parents. Besides informing them and asking for their permission, the letter stressed that their rejection would not affect the treatment of their child. It also provided the opportunity for parents to withdraw after having given their approval already. Also the clinicians were informed by a letter about their rights and about the fact that none of the footage would be used for the purpose of their individual assessment.

22   For an elaborate reflection on the need to start with a contextual exploration and without a camera, see Carroll and Mesman (2011).

23   See also Nugus et al., 2012 on the ethical requirements regarding participation in collaborative projects.

nurses in particular, do not work together during the same shift. Different forms were designed to inform each other on the topics to be filmed, what was already filmed, by whom and when, what footage was edited, which topics were discussed during which reflexivity meeting, etc. It was also decided that the team would come together for an all-day meeting four times a year to evaluate and, if needed, to re-organise things, as well as to discuss the next steps to be taken.

While the video team (including me) was using the video reflexivity method it was adjusted to the specificities of the neonatology ward. The video team designed an extensive infrastructure of communication. The team design a set of different forms in order to communicate between the members of the video team. In this way they could keep track of what was filmed, by whom, when and if it was already saved and edited. This infrastructure allowed for a smooth collaboration between the members of the video team who most of the time worked during different shifts. Besides the internal communication the team also made sure to tap in existing communication lines in order to inform both the nursing staff as the medical staff about the outcomes of the reflexivity meetings, like changes in ways of working. Two members of the team took up the responsibility to act as 'liaison officer', while someone else took up the role as chair or took care of the minutes of the meetings of the video team. With the development of forms and the assignment of roles and responsibilities the method was firmly situated in the particularities of the neonatology ward. On basis of experience the method was constantly refined in order to find the best fit to the ward's needs and dynamics. For example, the organisation of work (shifts and rotation) resulted in different teams every other week. To collect comments and suggestions from many colleagues it was decided to show the same footage for at least 10 weeks in order to discuss it with as many clinicians as possible. Additionally, the project was extended with the use of the video material for creating a visual aid to the written protocols for nursing care procedures. All these forms of contextualisation imply that the video reflexivity method did not only change practices on the ward, but was an object of change itself as well. Or to be more precise, the method has a flexibility that allows for tailor-made adjustments.[24]

The key players, such as the members of the video team and the other clinicians of the ward, are to be considered 'primary collaborators', meaning 'those who are clearly responsible because they have participated in defining the project and because they accept the project as valuable and as at least partially their responsibility' (Maeinschein, 1993: 171). But what about the 'secondary collaborators', those 'who contribute to the project but do not also fully participate in the project' (ibid.)?[25] Although they do not contribute directly, these non-users matter in their own way. Who were the secondary collaborators in the video reflexivity project?

---

24   This becomes very clear since I am involved in the introduction of the method on another ward.

25   Compare the weak and strong definition of collaboration of Katz and Martin (1997: 7).

How Non-Users Matter[26]

Since almost 80 per cent of the clinicians' work directly involves patients, following clinicians with a camera implies that patients appear on the video as well. Although they are not directly involved in the method, these non-users do matter. Regardless of the fact that they are too ill and too small to realise what is happening, their privacy is at stake. Therefore an informed consent of their parents, their legal representatives, was required and obtaining it was crucial. Unlike the clinical staff, the parents of NICU patients come and go (after a few days, a few weeks or, in exceptional cases, several months). This cohort of parents that is 'moving through' the ward needs to be informed about their role and rights as well. They were also guaranteed that refusal on their part would have no effect on their child's treatment. Although patients and parents do not actively participate in the project, they play a decisive role in the process of video reflexivity. Thus, it is crucial not only to have clinicians on your side, but also to convince the parents about the purpose of the project and the limited use of the footage. Some parents agreed instantly after explaining that the project was part of an internal patient safety improvement trajectory. Others were hesitant because they were not sure who would have access to the footage. Over time only a few parents refused, in most cases because they knew their baby was dying and in a few other cases because the timing proved unfortunate (when asked they were in complete stress because of their baby's sudden admission to the NICU). Later on in the project it was decided that parental consent would be asked during the official intake.

Who is considered to be involved is potentially an issue of dispute. This is not just a matter of 'taking a careful look around', but also, in the words of Hackett (2005), of the 'understandings of collaboration' (669). Collaborative activities are embedded in organisations with their own local power structures, policies and traditions. One should be aware of this while the social boundaries of the project are defined. For example, every project related to infection prevention should be discussed with the hospital's infection prevention officers. The fact that the project is an initiative of the ward does not make a difference. However, while we were setting up the collaborative texture everyone's focus was on the situation within the walls of the neonatology ward. One day one of the officers visited the ward while someone was filming. After being respectively surprised and upset she went to the head nurse to complain about not being informed about the project, which was underway for many months already. This example underscores the role of particular parties within the larger organisational structure, even if they do not take part directly in the collaborative activity as such.

---

26   This heading is inspired by Nelly Oudshoorn's and Trevor Pinch's *How Users Matter: The Co-Construction of Users and Technologies*. Cambridge, MA: The MIT Press, 2003.

Re-engineering Stages, Structures and Collaboration

In the previous section I described the establishment of a 'practice-improvement collaborative', discussing several aspects of collaboration such as the focus and the heterogeneity of the actors. Hackett (2005) has also indicated other dimensions of collaborative projects such as their intensity, velocity and output. These components refer to 'collaboration-in-action'. In the context of this chapter this raises the question of how the development of the video reflexivity project effects collaboration between the clinicians and my own role as actor. In this respect, the project was designed to make me superfluous. My position can be considered as a kind of 'planned obsolescence'. In order to hand over the ownership of the project, roles and responsibilities *had* to change. Although I had visions of gradual retreat, in the NICU practice gradualness does not exist. As will become clear below, health care practices, research practices and collaborative practices are strongly intertwined. To dissect this entanglement I discuss the development of the collaborative project and its velocity and intensity in particular. I will argue that collaboration is the outcome of a continuous co-construction of relations and internal re-engineering.

In practice the use of the video reflexivity method required a continuous 'internal reengineering' (Carise, Cornely and Gurel, 2002) to make the project fit the structure and workflow of the ward. Yet, the continuous reengineering had an effect on the collaboration. For instance, the official planning turned out to be completely useless and generated feelings of discomfort.

I anticipated the most intensive part of the project to take place in the first two months. By that time I expected to have trained the video team in how to select and edit video footage, as well as in chairing the reflexivity meetings' discussions. I had planned on spending the rest of the assigned time on anchoring the method on the ward by strengthening the support of the clinicians and the expertise of the video team. In this second stage my presence would not be required as often as in the first stage. However, this is not what happened. On the contrary, the first three months there was not a single day that allowed the clinicians to take the time to sit down and participate in a reflexivity meeting. Not one single day! During these months the NICU was overloaded and most of the patients were critically ill patients who required complex care and all the attention of the clinicians. While such a patient population provides many opportunities to film issues related to line infection, such as the insertion of a central catheter, the prolonged hectic circumstances on the NICU did not leave any window of opportunity to do something with this material.

The impossibility of organising reflexivity meetings influenced not only the velocity of my research output on patient safety (that is there were no reflexivity discussions to analyse), but also that of my collaboration with the clinicians. First, it resulted in an overall uneasiness. The clinicians felt uncomfortable that they could not make time for me, even though they strongly supported the project. Although there was no need for it, they apologised almost every day. I too felt uncomfortable because I was not able to show them anything while I had already been filming them for three months. This lack of time also revealed the assumptions that were implicitly written in the project's planning and structure. As if this critical care practice would allow room for an additional activity, such as filming colleagues, editing the video recordings and discussing the footage, without any compensation, or as if the workload on an NICU would be stable, no matter the number of admissions and the level of complexity of the patients. In other words, the whole setup of the project assumed a fixed stable practice that would open up easily to incorporate additional actions. In reality, however, the NICU practice is rigid in its structure and erratic in its workload. The moment I was about to give up and return my assignment to the management, the head-nurse saved the project by officially allocating time to the project. This decision was not initiated by a request of me, but based on their own frustration. The effect of this intervention was huge. Now at least the nurses of the video team had the opportunity to get actively engaged in the project.[27] Secondly, time and again the meetings were rescheduled until the best day of the week, time of day and place on the ward were found. It was important to avoid strong competition with other activities, like medical rounds or nursing observation rounds, because it would jeopardise the commitment of the clinicians, since these activities are at the heart of their professional duties. Thirdly, there was also no time for the members of the video team to learn how to film, edit and select the footage. This delay obstructed the transition of the project's 'ownership'; after three months it was still *my* project instead of theirs. My planned obsolescence concerning my own position seemed out of reach and thus the project appeared doomed. The allocation of time to the nurses to work on the project was crucial in order to shift the ownership. It had to become theirs in order to define it as a 'success'.

Part of the initial planning was based on some of my other responsibilities (for example teaching). These responsibilities could not be moved to another date. Now I had to leave the ward for some weeks while the project was not even in her first stage. In order to keep in touch, I did send emails to the members of the video team. Some of them read them and sometimes only after several days and I received just a few replies. During this time it became clear to me how different our professional cultures are. As a scholar I almost 'live in my mailbox' and its one of my main forms of communication. In this I differed from the members of the video team. Checking emails during working hours was not considered part of their job. Doing so might elicit responses from colleagues or even the parents while visiting their child. So, once in a while I went back to discuss matters face to face. It became immediately clear that the infrastructures of communication

---

27 Other changes that helped the project to survive concerned the frequency, day and time for the reflexivity meetings. It was decided to have weekly meetings. This would prevent the project from losing the attention of the clinicians when a meeting had to be cancelled due to lack of time. Now it would only take a week until the next possibility for a meeting would occur.

within the team should not be based on email exchange. Instead a folder with forms was created.

The three months of delay also created some unforeseen changes in the distribution of roles and responsibilities. Part of the initial planning was based on some of my other responsibilities (for example teaching) that could not be moved to another date. Due to these obligations for some weeks I had no time to be on the ward. Yet, my compelling teaching schedule turned out to be a blessing in disguise as it had a very positive effect on both the project and the collaboration between the video team and myself. During my absence the video team became very active and made the project theirs. Instead of me, now they took care of all the arrangements and practicalities required to maintain the project. For example, the meetings were chaired by one of them and they had developed all kinds of forms and procedures for communication within the team as well as with their medical and nursing colleagues on the ward.[28] The collaboration had moved from me being on the one side (a researcher who tried to do 'her thing') and the ward/video team on the other side, meanwhile reaching out towards each other on the basis of our good intentions, to a situation of being one team in which we all shared the hope that there would be enough time for a meeting, the joy if it worked out well and the frustration if it didn't. Sharing our ambitions, commitments and, perhaps even more so, frustrations turned out to be strong social glue.[29] My absence, as it turned out, had not hindered the project. On the contrary, it created room for a re-distribution of roles and responsibilities, which in its own way benefited the effectiveness of the project. It is only in hindsight that we can judge whether particular situations or certain developments are opportunities or obstacles for collaboration.

The processes described above demonstrate the entanglement of health care practices, research practices and collaborative practice. Collaboration is always a contextualised collaboration. Whereas most studies on collaboration understandably highlight the importance of the organisational context in which the collaboration takes place (for example Nugus et al., 2012), I prefer a wider focus. In other words, not only the organisation where the project is located is a factor of influence. The context that influences the relationship between the participants is constituted by all involved organisations. Both the NICU, with its fluctuating number and complexity of admissions and corresponding workload, and the university with its academic calendar bring in their own institutional ecologies that constitute a specific framework that affects the velocity and intensity of the collaborative processes in the video project.

---

28   This dramatic change also underlined the fact that one's intensive presence will not always contribute to the progress of a project, but instead may leave no room for others to act.

29   Needless to say that joining the competition *and* winning the Patient Safety Prize 2012 of the hospital also contributed to the teambuilding.

The Collaborative Space: A Stone in the Pond

After some time the socio-geographical space in which the method was used expanded beyond the walls of the neonatology ward. The video team realised that filming on the NICU was not enough to capture the issue of infection prevention and the insertion of a line in particular. It also required, for example, filming in the surgery department where the patients are handed over after being born by a Caesarean. Also here the neonatology team had to act safely. Likewise their presence in the delivery room required the attention of the video camera. In other words, the need to follow NICU doctors and nurses is not limited to the neonatology ward but is extended to other parts of the hospital as well.

Moreover, the video project on the neonatology ward unexpectedly catalysed all kinds of new collaborations. First, it resulted in collaboration with the Midwifery Department. Some of their researchers asked me to join their brainstorm session for a research project on communication and collaboration between midwives and obstetricians. Together we designed a PhD project on this topic in which video reflexivity sessions with midwifes and obstetricians, as well as sessions that also include parents (to be), act as the core method of data collection. Furthermore, the project also had a focus on why communication and collaboration went well while the notion of exnovation was one of the central concepts. Secondly, due to the video project on the NICU I became involved in the supervision of a bachelor thesis for a programme at one of the Belgian universities of applied sciences at the other side of the border. It was one of the NICU nurses on the video team who proposed to use the footage as a visual aid to the protocols. By using a hyperlink nurses could *see* how to do the procedure correctly. While this idea was very positively received on the ward, she also turned it into a research topic as part of her Bachelor training in order to become a manager of care and I was asked to act as her local supervisor. Thirdly, the neighbouring ward, Paediatrics, also showed an interest in video reflexivity. After some exploratory talks and a presentation to the team the first contours of a second video team are emerging. It was decided that I would train them on how to use this method, implying that I will spend considerable time on the paediatric ward and the Paediatric intensive care unit (PICU). Fourthly, I started to collaborate with one of the researchers from the Quality and Safety Division of the hospital. We met on a 'fair' organised by the hospital where everyone could display his or her good ideas for patient safety as part of a contest for the 'best idea on patient safety' (which we won). She was impressed by the video reflexivity method but criticised the fact that we did not measure its impact. Realising she was right I contacted her afterwards and now we are working together with the aim to find a way to get the required resources for an extensive project that concentrates on the video reflexivity method as object of analysis. What started as a collaborative project on the neonatology ward linked me up with the Department of Midwifery, the Paediatric Department, the Department of Quality and Safety and a Belgian university of Applied Science. Collaboration never comes alone. Instead, it opens doors and creates passageways in which the involved parties can travel in both directions.

Collaboration, it turns out, may well act as a self-replicating phenomenon. Before you know it, you are entangled in a web of commitments, multiple ambitions, fine-tuning, choices and decisions, as well as expectations, (potential) disappointments and satisfaction. The growth of collaborative engagements also exemplifies their resourcefulness. The strength of collaboration has turned it into an almost undisputed way of organising work. However, collaboration, as I will discuss in the final section, always requires a valuation of its necessity.

Concluding Remarks

Zittoun et al. (2007) has stressed how working together can generate two different kinds of knowledge: scientific knowledge and collaborative knowledge. This book, including this chapter, focuses on the latter kind. In the previous sections I reflected on my boundary-spanning engagement with the neonatal ward. These reflections made me realise the amount of years I spent on the NICU *without* collaborating with the clinicians. This all changed due to the method of video reflexivity that acted as an infrastructure for collaboration. Without the method I was probably still on the ward, but just doing 'my own business'. In this way the video reflexivity method acted as a form of 'pragmatic trial' (Janssen, 2012). Pragmatic trials provide an infrastructure for the implementation of change based on collaboration between the researcher and the practitioners.[30] In other words, the method of video reflexivity enabled me to change my identity from an individual researcher into a team member of the ward. It enabled me to learn *together* with the people I had studied for so many years, about NICU practice.

The reflections in this chapter made me also aware how similar and different we are in our ambitions. My collaboration with the neonatology staff was motivated by multiple reasons and concerns of a quite different nature, such as epistemological curiosity, safety concerns, emancipatory intentions as well as patient care, power structures and quality improvement. They are related to my research project and their work environment, to the patients in the hospital and the professionals who take care of them. To achieve our ambitions we work together. Zittoun et al. (2007) considers collaboration as a system of development (210). To approach 'collaboration' as a system they stress the dynamical character. Things change in the collaboration and may lead to new practices, new relationships, new goals and new perspectives (212). In other words, collaboration has concrete effects. This implies that collaboration is also a form

---

30   Pragmatic trials can be considered as evaluation studies that are adjusted to the specificities of particular daily practices of care. Being critical about the pragmatic level of the existing trials, Janssen (2012) pleas for more pragmatism in order to close the gap between the evaluation of practices and the practices themselves.

of intervention. By definition, according to Zuiderent-Jerak and Jensen (2007), intervention does not mean one-way causation, but should be considered a form of 'artful contamination' (231) that takes place in a hybrid space in which all involved parties are subjected to the forces of interaction. From this perspective collaboration becomes a form of opening up and allowing intrusion on different levels: agenda setting, and distribution of tasks, responsibility and credits, just to name a few. Caswill and Shove (2000) have pointed out that collaboration is not free of dangers. For example, as described in the third section, my agenda only partly overlapped with those of the neonatology ward. This in itself didn't have to be a problem. Nevertheless, there is always the risk of one's research agenda being appropriated by other actors. When is 'giving in and being flexible' becoming a threat to one's own ambitions? There is the danger of co-optation, including the risk of ending up playing no significant role and losing every space for genuine research and interaction.[31] Can close collaboration with the clinicians result in the abandonment of my research aspirations or in getting aligned with sheer managerial agendas? How can I prevent my project from evolving beyond recognition? Instead of answering these questions I would like to call attention to the issue of collaboration itself.[32]

Some authors, like Morse (2008), advocate a more critical stance towards collaboration, especially in the area of qualitative research. Nowadays, according to Morse, team research is fast becoming the key to successful grant applications (3). Morse's worries about this development concern qualitative research in particular. Her worry is that research assistants (RA) will collect the data while the principal investigator (PI) will do the analysis. In these cases the contextual knowledge, which is essential to be able to analyse the data properly, will get lost in the transition from RA to PI. This is a concern about the quality of qualitative research projects. Although my collaborative work with the clinicians worked out very well for both sides, I acknowledge Janice Morse's plea to reflect on collaboration beyond the standard questions of how, with whom and about what. But instead we first need to focus on questions about why to collaborate and its consequences for data collection and analysis and the wider research context. There seems to be a tendency simply to ignore the question of whether there is actually a need to collaborate. Cheek (2008) even refers to 'an imperative to collaborate' (1599). The well-known phrase 'publish or perish' might soon be replaced by 'partnership or perish' (ibid.). Notwithstanding this plea for caution in order not to fall into the trap of 'collaborating solely for the purpose of being involved into collaboration', this chapter testifies how collaboration between different parties can result in a structural practice improvement. This improvement could not have been accomplished without the active engagement of all actors involved.

---

31   For the different possible positions in intervening, see Downey and Dumit (1997).
32   For an attempt to answer these questions, see Mesman (2007).

References

Amabile, T.A., Patterson, C., Mueller, J., Wojcik, T., Odomirok, P.W., Marsh, M. and Kramer, S.J. 2001. Academic–practitioner collaboration in management research: A case of cross-profession collaboration. *The Academy of Management Journal*, 44(2), 418–31.

Carise, D., Cornely, W., Gurel, O. 2002. A successful researcher practitioner collaboration in substance abuse treatment. *Journal of Substance Abuse Treatment*, 23, 157–62.

Carroll, K., Iedema, I. and Kerridge, R. 2008. Reshaping ICU ward round practices using video-reflexive ethnography. *Qualitative Health Research*, 18(3), 380–90.

Carroll, K. 2009. Insider, outsider, alongsider: Examining reflexivity in hospital-based video research. *International Journal of Multiple Research Approaches*, 3(3), 246–63.

Carroll, K. and Mesman, J. 2011. Ethnographic context meets ethnographic biography: A challenge for the mores of doing fieldwork. *International Journal of Methodological Research Approaches*, 5, 155–68.

Caswill, Ch. and Shove, E. 2000. Introducing interactive social science. *Science and Public Policy*, 27(3), 154–8.

Cheek, J. 2008. Researching collaboratively: Implications for qualitative research and researchers. *Qualitative Health Research*, 18, 1599.

Clark, C., Moss, P.A., Goering, S., Herter, R.J., Lamar, B., Leonard, D., Robbins, S., Russell, M., Templin, M. and Wascha, K. 1996. Collaboration as a dialogue: Teachers and researchers engaged in conversation and professional development. *American Educational Research Journal*, 33(1), 193–231.

Dooner, A.M., Mandzuk, D. and Clifton, R.A. 2008. Stages of collaboration and the realities of professional learning communities. *Teaching and Teacher Education*, 24, 564–74.

Downey, G.L. and Dumit, J. 1997. Locating and intervening: An introduction. In: G.L. Downey and J. Dumit (eds) *Cyborgs and Citadels. Anthropological interventions in Emerging Sciences and Technologies.* Santa Fe: School of American Press, 5–11.

Downey, G.L. 2009. What is engineering studies for? Dominant practices and scalable scholarship. *Engineering Studies*, 1(1), 55–76.

Fortun, K. and Cherkasky, T. 1998. Counter-expertise and the politics of collaboration. *Science as Culture*, 7(2), 145–72.

Hackett, E.J. 2005. Introduction: Special guest-edited issue on scientific collaboration. *Social Studies of Science*, 35(5), 667–71.

Iedema, R. and Carroll, K. 2011. The 'clinalyst': Institutionalizing reflexive space to realize safety and flexible systematization in health care. *Journal of Organizational Change Management*, 24(2): 175–90.

Iedema, R., Long, D., Forsyth, R. and Bosnan Lee, B. 2006. Visibilising clinical work: Video ethnography in the contemporary hospital. *Health Sociology Review*, 15, 156–68.

Iedema, R. and Merrick, E. 2008. *HELiCS: Handover-Enabling Learning in Communication for Safety.* Australian Commission on Safety and Quality in Health Care and the University of Technology, Sydney.

Iedema, R., Mesman, J. and Carroll, K. 2013. *Visualising Health Care Practice Improvement: Innovation from Within.* London: Radcliffe Publishing.

Jansen, Y.J.F.M. 2012. *Pragmatic Trials: The Mutual Shaping of Research and Primary Health Care Practice.* Doctoral thesis, Erasmus University, Rotterdam, the Netherlands.

Katz, J.S. and Martin, B.R. 1997. What is research collaboration? *Research Policy*, 26(1), 1–18.

Lasker, R.D., Weiss, E.S. and Miller, R. 2001. Partnership synergy: A practical framework for studying and strengthening the collaborative advantage. *The Milbank Quarterly*, 79(2), 179–205.

Latour, B. 1992. Where are the missing masses? The sociology of a few mundane artifacts. In: W.E. Bijker and J. Law (eds) *Shaping Technology/ Building Society: Studies in Sociotechnical Change.* Cambridge, MA: The MIT, 225–58.

Lynch, M. 2009. Science as a vacation: Deficits, surfeits, PUSS, and doing your own job. *Organization*, 16(1), 101–19.

Maienschein, J. 1993. Why collaborate. *Journal of History of Biology*, 26(2), 167–83.

Mesman, J. 2007. Disturbing observations as a basis for collaborative research. *Science as Culture, Special Issue: Unpacking 'Intervention' in STS*, (16)3, 281–95.

Mesman, J. 2008. *Uncertainty in Medical Innovation: Experienced Pioneers in Neonatal Care.* Hampshire: Palgrave MacMillan.

Mesman J. 2010. Diagnostic work in collaborative practices in neonatal care. In: M. Büscher, D. Goodwin and J. Mesman (eds) *Ethnographies of Diagnostic Work: Dimensions of Transformative Practice.* Palgrave Macmillan, 140–66.

Mesman, J. 2012a. Resources of strength: An exnovation of hidden competences to preserve patient safety. In: E. Rowley and J. Waring (eds) *A Socio-Cultural Perspective on Patient Safety.* Aldershot: Ashgate Publishing Ltd., 72–92.

Mesman, J. 2012b. Moving in with care: About patient safety as a spatial achievement. *Space and Culture*, 15(1), 31–43.

Morris, N. and Hebden, J.C. 2008. Evolving collaborations: A self-referential case-study of a social/natural sciences collaborative project. *Science Studies*, 21(2), 27–46.

Morse, J.M. 2008. Styles of collaboration in qualitative inquiry. *Qualitative Health Research*, 18(3), 3–4.

Nugus, P., Greenfield, D., Travaglia, J. and Braithwaite, J. 2012. The politics of action research: 'If you don't like the way things are going, get off the bus'. *Social Science and Medicine*, 75, 1946–53.

Oudshoorn, N. and Pinch, T. 2003. *How Users Matter: The Co-Construction of Users and Technologies.* Cambridge, MA: The MIT Press.

Owen, C., Wackers, G. and Béguin, P. (eds) 2009. *Risky Work Environments. Reappraising Human Work with-in Fallible Systems.* Aldershot: Ashgate.

Parker, J., Vermeulen, N. and Penders, B. (eds) 2010. *Collaboration in the New Life Sciences.* Aldershot: Ashgate.

Paulus, T.M., Woodside, M. and Ziegler, M.F. 2010. 'I tell you, it's a journey, isn't it?' Understanding collaborative meaning making in qualitative research. *Qualitative Inquiry,* 16(10), 852–62.

Penders, B. and Radstake, M. (forthcoming). Critique in action: Assembling shared matters of concern with corporate R&D. Working paper.

Pinch, T., Collins, H.M. and Carbone, L. 1996. Inside knowledge: Second order measures of skill. *The Sociological Review,* 44(2), 163–86.

Reeves, S., Lewin, S., Espin, S. and Zwarenstein, M. 2010. *Interprofessional Teamwork for Health and Social Care.* San Francisco, CA: Wiley-Blackwell.

Rizzo, M. 2005. Striving to eliminate catheter-related bloodstream infections: A literature review of evidence-based strategies. *Seminars in Anesthesia,* 24, 214–25.

Roper, L. 2001. Achieving successful academic–practitioner research collaboration. *Development in Practice,* 12(3/4), 338–454.

Rubinson, L. and Diette, G. 2004. Best practices for insertion of central venous catheters in intensive-care units to prevent catheter-related bloodstream infections. *The Journal of Laboratory and Clinical Medicine,* 143, 5–13.

Sheretz, R.J., Wesley Ely, E., Westbrook, D.M., Gledhill, K.S., Streed, S.A., Kiger, B., et al. 2000. Education of physicians-in-training can decrease the risk for vascular catheter infection. *Annals of Internal Medicine,* 132, 641–8.

Shrum, W., Chompalov, I. and Genuth, J. 2001. Trust, conflict and performance in scientific collaborations. *Social Studies of Science,* 31(5), 681–730.

Shrum, W., Genuth, J., and Chompalov, I. 2007. *Structures of Scientific Collaboration.* Cambridge, MA: The MIT Press.

Star, S.L. 1991b. The sociology of the invisible: The primacy of work in the writings of Anselm Strauss. In: D.R. Maines (ed.) *Social Organization and Social Process: Essays in Honor of Anselm Strauss.* Hawthorne: Aldine de Gruyter, 265–83.

Weick, K.E. 1979. *The Social Psychology of Organizing.* Reading, MA: Addison-Wesley.

Wilde de, R. 2000. Innovating innovation: A contribution to the philosophy of the future. Keynote at *Policy Agendas for Sustainable Technological Innovation.* London, 2 December 2000.

Zittoun, T., Baucal, A., Cornish, F. and Gillespie, A. 2007. Collaborative research, knowledge and emergence. *Integrative Psychological and Behavioral Science,* 41, 208–17.

Zuiderent-Jerak, T. 2007. Preventing implementation: Exploring interventions with standardization in healthcare. *Science as Culture,* 16(3), 311–29.

Zuiderent-Jerak, T. and Jensen, C.B. 2007. Editorial introduction: Unpacking 'intervention' in science and technology studies. *Science as Culture,* 16(3), 227–35.

Chapter 10

Health Care Collaboration Between Patients and Physicians

Benjamin Lewin

The interactions that occur between patients and physicians during medical visits are an essential point for the enactment of health care. The aim of this chapter is to bring attention to the role that patients play, as collaborative agents, during interactions with physicians in the practice of health care. While some chapters in this book have discussed collaboration in health care, as opposed to collaboration in health research, the collaborative potential of *individual* patients in the context of health care settings has yet to be explored. The lack of attention to patients in the context of health care at the interactional level is reflected in the STS literature outside of this book as well. The invisibility of patients as collaborative agents in STS literature leads to the conclusion, intended or not, that the patients are passive recipients of medical care. This is reflective of a larger cultural phenomenon that has its roots in the professional dominance of medical experts (Starr, 1984).

Traditionally, much of the literature on scientific collaboration that came from STS and neighboring disciplines focused on collaboration between professionals. However, Stephen Epstein (2008) notes that since 1990, the study of public participation in medicine has "mushroomed." This observation is noted in a chapter of the third edition of *The Handbook of Science and Technology Studies*, which includes an entire section on "Politics and Publics." Although the handbook is not limited in scope to medical research, this section does include substantial discussion related to public participation in medicine. In the same section of this handbook, Bucchi and Neresini (2008) define public participation as, "the diversified set of situations and activities ... whereby nonexperts become involved, and provide their own input to, agenda setting, decision-making, policy forming, and knowledge production processes regarding science" (p. 449). It is clear that they had macro-processes in mind when conceptualizing the role of the public (nonexperts). Phrases such as "agenda setting" and "policy forming" are suggestive of social movements and nonexpert interest groups. The focus on large-scale phenomena is coupled with a focus on aggregates instead of individuals in the STS literature. Epstein (2008) explains the increased attention to patient groups and health movements as a result of numerous factors: 1) Patient groups and health movements have become more prolific over the last few decades. 2) There is also more literature on the subject because STS has expanded its focus beyond traditional laboratory settings. 3) Also, increased attention to health and illness. The expansion of biomedicine into more areas of politics, daily life, and science also explains the surge in STS literature on health movements and patient groups. Although public participation in the field of medicine has been examined in the context of social groups and movements, the same cannot be said for interactional, micro-processes. Health care includes not only the politics and knowledge production of health and illness influenced by social movements, but it also includes the day-to-day practice of medicine at the interactional level. So how is it, then, that the collaborative potential of individual patients has been overlooked in STS literature?

The relative lack of attention to patients in STS research on collaboration is understandable given the history of the discipline and current conceptions of what it means to collaborate. A likely explanation for the lack of attention of patients in STS research on medical collaboration is rooted in the ways in which collaboration is conceptualized. Early research on collaboration usually equated collaborative work to coauthored publications. This was a common metric, despite the fact that researchers recognized the problems that arose with such a simple operationalization of a quite complex phenomenon (Subramanyam, 1983). Following the call by Katz and Martin (1997) for a more nuanced conceptualization of collaboration, researchers began to move beyond simple bibliometric analysis and explore other ways to operationalize collaborative work. Katz and Martin (1997) recognized the "fuzzy or ill-defined border" that exists in trying to identify the boundary of collaboration. While acknowledging the variability of the location of the border around collaboration, the authors specifically state that, "the group of collaborators will generally exclude ... those not seen as, or treated as, 'proper' researchers" (p. 8). Technicians and research assistants are included in this definition, but using this criterion to define the borders of collaborative work would certainly exclude nonexperts, such as patients.

The focus on research, as opposed to care, coupled with a focus on "proper" researchers all but excludes patients as collaborators. Hackett (2005) acknowledges the complexity of understanding the "*heterogeneity*, or the variety of participants, purposes ... and modalities of collaboration" (italics added, p. 669). A new variety of participant—the individual patient, and a new modality—health care, as opposed to health research, are presented in this chapter. The theories and concepts, mostly stemming from the field of medical sociology, are not meant to be an exhaustive review of sociological literature on patient collaboration. Instead, high profile theories and concepts are synthesized in order to provide readers who may not otherwise be exposed to this body of literature an opportunity to think about patients as collaborative agents in health care processes.

Low-collaboration Models of Physician–Patient Interaction

Interaction is necessary, but not sufficient for collaboration. Interactions are communications between two or more people. Collaboration involves cooperative work toward some specific objective—in this case, optimal patient health. As the following two subsections demonstrate, physicians and patients can interact, and move toward the objective of patient health, but may do so in a way that has a low degree of cooperation. There are numerous models to explain interactions between the physician and patient, some which include very low levels of collaboration. An example of a low-collaboration interaction would be something as simple as a patient stating a symptom list with no other input during the physician visit. Models of physician–patient interaction are distributed along a continuum of power within the physician–patient interaction ranging from high levels of physician control and agency at one end of the spectrum to high levels of patient control and agency at the other end. This continuum of power has been the primary axis upon which theorists have situated their models of physician–patient interaction. While different authors have introduced many models along this continuum, they can be classified within three main categories—the two ends of the power spectrum and a middle ground which positions both the physician and the patient as exercising equal degrees of power within the interaction. After covering the non-collaborative models of interaction, I will move to a discussion of the "middle ground" models of interaction that allow for physician–patient collaboration.

Physician-centered Interactions

The oldest sociological models of physician–patient interaction date back to the 1950s. Given the historical context in which the early models of interaction were formulated, it is no surprise that they position the physician as the central figure in the interaction while the patient is almost invisible, except as a recipient of medical expertise and action. Early models that were built around high degrees of physician authority were formed during the "golden age of doctoring" (McKinlay and Marceau, 2002), which resulted in unprecedented degrees of professional dominance (Starr, 1984). The most popular sociological model during the 1950s and into the 1960s was that of Talcott Parsons (1951), who presents a relationship in which the physician maintains an "affect-neutral" association with the patient. Such relationships have little emotional involvement, creating an instrumental dialog between physician and patient. According to Parsons, this "affect-neutral" relationship stems from the norms and role expectations that surround both parties. Because illness of any type is considered a negative, undesirable state in this model, patients are expected to understand and comply with the norms set forth by the sick role. Under the two conditions that the patient 1) wants to improve his/her health and return to a normal functioning member of society and 2) the patient will seek the help of a legitimized authority figure (i.e. physician), the patient is granted entry into the sick role. Upon legitimate entry into the sick role, he/she is 1) not held responsible for the illness and 2) exempt from normal social obligations until recovery. The physician's role in this relationship is to legitimize the patient's claim of disease and to provide adequate treatment for the given illness.

Despite Parsons' description of the physician–patient relationship as affect-neutral, he also draws a direct comparison with the parent–child relationship. While most parents do not have an affect-neutral relationship with their children, the association does provide a vivid metaphor. Just like a father instructing his son on proper behavior in specific situations, the physician, with the interest of the patient in mind, uses his professional knowledge to command the patient. The patient, just like the son, is dependent and expected to listen and follow directions given by the authority figure. Because of this commonly used comparison, this Parsonian model of the physician–patient relationship is often referred to as the paternalistic model. In this model, patient agency is restricted to giving consent to whatever treatment the physician feels is best (Emanuel, 2000).

Parsons' conceptualization of the physician–patient relationship has received a great deal of criticism. One common critique of this model is that it is not easily applied to chronic illnesses. While those patients with acute illness can be exempt from social obligations for a short period of time, those who have a chronic condition may not be able to avoid social obligations forever. Another familiar critique of this model is that disease is a social construction, and therefore the reality of disease is defined and shaped by the current zeitgeist. Depending on the current norms and values of society, illnesses sometimes fall under the responsibility of the individual. For example, the sick individual is not held responsible for her malady when she has the flu, but a man who is obese and suffers from heart disease is often blamed for his condition. When the individual is forced to take blame for his or her disease, they no longer are allowed the social exemptions associated with the sick role.

Szasz and Hollender (1956) offer a modified theory of physician–patient relationships that accounts for disease type. Where Parsons fails to account for chronic illness, Szasz and Hollender propose that the amount of patient participation is dependent on the illness being treated. When dealing with acute illness, patients take a passive role in the medical process. As the disease moves from acute to chronic, the patient becomes more active in the treatment process while the physician moves from an assertive authority to a guiding authority. In all cases, the patient is still viewed as dependent on the expertise of the physician, but those patients with chronic diseases take the most active role in treatment (Szasz and Hollender, 1956). The understanding that disease type may influence interaction dynamics hints at a continuum of power and agency between physicians and patients; patient passivity is not a fixed feature of the physician–patient relationship. To be sure, the paternalistic, physician-centered model is still a valid descriptor of many interactions. This, paired with the traditional focus of STS on research and experts, may explain the invisibility of patients as collaborative agents in STS literature.

Patient-centered Interactions

At the other end of the power spectrum, patients control the interaction and decisions that emerge from it. While names vary, all models on this end of the spectrum are founded on the premise that patients act as autonomous agents in determining their own treatment outcomes. One of the earlier conceptualizations of this power dynamic is referred to as the consumer model. The consumer model reframes the patient as a health care consumer instead of a dependent patient. Reeder (1972) was one of the first to recognize the change in physician–patient interaction and to describe a type of relationship that emerged from the consumer rights movement of the 1960s. Whereas in the paternalistic model, the patient is expected to adhere to the orders of the physician, in the consumer model, the patient acts as an autonomous agent, selectively using advice of one or more physicians to help make informed decisions. Haug and Lavin (1981) conceive of the consumer model of physician–patient interaction as an exchange relationship. Public movements and legal legislation such as the Patients' Bill of Rights reflect the popular idea that health care relationships should be framed as a client–provider interaction instead of the authoritative relationship found in the paternalistic model. This consumer model is rather straightforward in that the patient is seen as the consumer of a product, while the doctor supplies the patient with the desired commodity. Because the patient is dependent upon correct and appropriate information from the physician to make informed decisions, the relationship becomes somewhat fiduciary, like that of a client–provider relationship. Just as providers of other goods and services are expected to uphold a level of fairness and integrity, so are physicians. This model views the physician–patient interaction through the lens of exchange market philosophies. Viewing physician–patient interaction through this consumerist oriented lens, the patient (consumer) is seen as having high autonomy.

It should be noted that while parallels can be made between the consumption of health care and the consumption of other goods and services, there are fundamental differences. Ultimately, patients still depend on the professional authority of physicians so that they may legitimately enter the sick role. The physician acts at gatekeeper to the sick role; other consumer–supplier relationships do not have this type of power dynamic. Patients cannot claim exemption from daily obligations based on a self-diagnosed disease. Much like our old elementary school days, eventually the teacher (or employer, or family member) will want to see a "letter from the doctor." Another fundamental difference between the consumption of health care and the consumption of most of the goods and services is the monopoly that physicians hold on medical knowledge. Despite this dependency on physicians for legitimacy and knowledge, the consumer model is still relevant in that physicians provide information so that patients may make informed decisions. The physician then authorizes the patient's decision so that the patient may then be granted legitimacy by a medical professional. At the heart of this model lies a consumer who (through the help of the physician) makes an informed decision.

Another iteration of the high patient-centered model is referred to as both the informed decision-making model and the evidence-based patient choice model. This model is characterized by the physician providing the patient with relevant information regarding his or her situation and then the patient being the active agent in deliberations and decision-making

(Hope, 1999; Charles, Gafni and Whelan, 1999). As argued by Charles, Gafni, and Whelan (1997), the decision-making process lies solely in the hands of the patient. It is true that the physician plays an active role through the dissemination of information, but once the patient has received that information, the physician becomes a passive agent. These patient-centered models of interaction may suggest some degree of collaboration due to a transfer of knowledge and a subsequent decision based upon that knowledge. However, because the actual decision-making process resides solely within the patient, these models are only superficially collaborative; the physician is nothing more than a medium for delivery of expert knowledge. This model differs slightly from the consumer model in that the impetus for this conceptualization is based on patient rights, as opposed to consumer market models of power. Emphasis on patient choice stems from the ethical belief that patients will have different preferences based on their personal value systems and that treatment decisions should be made by the individual who will undertake the treatment (Hope, 1999; Ford, Schofield and Hope, 2003).

Ultimately, decision-making in a clinical context rests upon the fusion of two distinct elements—information and preferences (Charles, Gafni and Whelan, 1997; Sebban et al., 1995; Levine et al., 1992). Professional and scientific information resides within the physician, while personal preferences regarding the experience and outcomes of treatment options reside within the patient. So far, I have described interactional models at each end of this axis of agency. The refocusing of agency that occurs with a shift from a paternalistic to a consumer model of interaction results in increased attention to patient autonomy and agency, thus allowing for a multi-directional flow of information, suggestions, and instructions between physicians and patients. This increased agency allows patients to take an active role in both the diagnostic process and in making decisions about treatments. But what does this fully collaborative model look like?

High-collaboration Models of Physician–Patient Interaction

While the paternalistic and consumer models describe each end of previously described continuum of power of physician–patient autonomy, there is a middle ground. Calls for this type of interaction can be dated back to the early 1970s (Veatch, 1972). This "collaborative sweet spot" is sometimes referred to as the shared decision-making model. Using the term "models" may be more appropriate given the multitude of ways in which this type of interaction is framed. Despite some differences in these models, they are all clustered near the center of the physician–patient power continuum. While there may not be explicit debate in the literature between competing models, consensus has yet to be reached as to what exactly is meant by shared decision-making. The fact that there are a multitude of names for this type of collaborative work between patients and physicians is suggestive of this lack of collective conceptualization. Models such as "enhanced autonomy" (Chin, 2002; Quill and Brody, 1996), "evidence-based patient choice" (Eysenbach and Jadad, 2001; Ford, Schofield and Hope, 2003), and "concordance" (Marinker and Sharp, 1997; Bissell, May and Noyce, 2004), among others, vary in some degree as to their particular points of exploration and emphasis. In an attempt to integrate these varied models, Makoul and Clayman (2006) examined 418 articles on shared decision-making and found that 61.5 percent of them mentioned shared decision-making without operationalizing it. Of the articles that did provide a conceptual definition, they found 31 distinct concepts used to describe shared decision-making. Of these, only two ("patient values/preferences" and "options") were found in at least half of the definitions. Although the conceptualization of these models may not be analogous, it does not mean that they are entirely disparate in their descriptions of power dynamics. The underlying theme that connects all of these models is that they involve a process in which information, values, preferences, and deliberations are shared between the patient and physician. This collective knowledge is then used by both parties to come to a mutually agreed-upon course of action. This is fundamentally different from the physician-centered model in which the physician makes all decisions with minimal input from the patient or the patient-based model in which the opposite holds true.

Collaborating on Treatment Decisions: Shared Decision Making

Two separate studies (Makoul and Clayman, 2006; Moumjid et al., 2007) found that the most frequently cited definition of shared decision-making comes from Charles et al. (1997; 1999). In this conceptualization, collaboration is framed within the context of making decisions specific to treatment (i.e. a diagnosis has already been assigned). Charles et al. (1999) note the variety of situations and contexts in which decision making occurs, but apply their model to treatment decisions that revolve around potentially life-threating diseases, such as early stage breast cancer. The focus is on diseases that involve "key treatment decision points which may occur only once and arise early on in the course of the disease which have major consequences for the patient" (p. 682). They argue that understanding shared decision making is essential in this context:

> ... first, because several treatment options exist with different possible outcomes, and substantial uncertainty. Second, there is often no clear-cut right or wrong answer. Third, treatments will vary in their impact on the patient's physical and psychological well-being ...

Within this context, the decision making process can be divided into three distinct stages. Charles et al. (1999) note that these "are analytically distinct stages, even though, in reality, these may occur together or in an iterative process" (p. 654).

During the first stage, information exchange, the patient shares self-knowledge while the physician shares technical knowledge. Keep in mind that the information exchange occurs within the context of an already diagnosed disease. Information such as patient health history and symptom severity is still important in that they may direct treatment options. The patient may not only reveal symptoms, health history, and contextualizing factors regarding health issues, but may also inform the physician about his medical knowledge related to the problem at hand. In this stage the physician will inform the patient about any relevant medical knowledge including treatment options and risks and benefits associated with these options. The second analytic stage, deliberation, focuses on communicating treatment preferences. For Charles and colleagues (1999), the key element to this stage is its "interactional nature." In this stage, collaboration is extended beyond information exchange to an expression of preferences. In the traditional, Parsonian physician-centered model, the doctor deliberates on the proper course of treatment without preferential input form the patient. Counter to this, in the patient-centered model, the patient is solely responsible for deliberation. An exchange between the patient and physician regarding treatment preferences may be affable or contentious, depending on whether or not the patient and physician are in agreement regarding the course of action for treatment. If there is disagreement, negotiation and bargaining may take place. The third analytic stage involves the actual act of making a treatment decision. Charles et al. (1999) provide little detail on this final stage other than to contrast it to the paternalistic and the informed choice models. In contrast to the non-collaborative models in which either the physician (paternalistic model) or patient (informed choice model) is solely responsible for making final treatment decisions, the shared decision model is the only one of the three in which the actual treatment decision is shared by the patient and physician.

It should be emphasized that in all three stages, both parties make contributions to the collaborative process. "Both patients and physicians bring both information and values; it is not simply a question of physicians bringing knowledge and patients bringing values" (Charles, Gafni and Whelan, 1997: 687). Patients bring knowledge not only in the form of symptoms and physiological experiences, but also knowledge about the lived, subjective experience of an illness. Within the context of a larger value system, the lived experience of a particular illness may influence beliefs about treatment. The decision to proceed with therapies that significantly reduce quality of life (such as radiation therapy and chemotherapy) is weighed against the (sometimes slim) chance of prolonging life. In situations like these, patient values become an important part of the collaborative process. While the physician brings expert knowledge to the encounter, he or she is also guided by a set of values and beliefs that may dictate how information is communicated and what treatment options are divulged or emphasized. One rather obvious example is the impact of a physician's religious beliefs on reproductive issues and the impact that those religious beliefs have on shaping the way a physician presents (or omits) possible treatment options to patients.

As is true with any form of collaboration, conflict may arise regarding the best course of action for the involved parties. Given the professional authority of the physician and the need for the sick role (and corresponding treatments) to be legitimated by a medical expert, it is easy to assume that the patient must submit to the will of the physician. However, physicians increasingly report feeling pressure to acquiesce to patient preferences. Decreased patient satisfaction can lead to patients moving from one practice to another, otherwise known as "doctor shopping" (Safran et al., 2001; Kasteler et al., 1976). Physicians are well aware that patients are willing to leave a doctor to find another whose medical opinions align with their own and are increasingly willing to capitulate to patient demands. For example, when patients make a drug request that was prompted by a pharmaceutical advertisement, over half of the physicians who wrote a prescription report that they did so partly to accommodate the patient's request. Of these physicians who fulfilled the patient's request for the advertised drug, five percent report doing so despite the fact that they believe a different drug our treatment was more appropriate (Weissman et al., 2004). These statistics reveal the degree to which physicians feel pressure to comply with patient requests.

When disagreement about the proper treatment path does arise, patients and physicians must find a resolution. Hayes-Bautista (1976) outlines the bargaining process between the patient and the physician regarding forms of treatment. Patients use a number of "convincing tactics" such as 1) demands, 2) suggestions, and 3) leading questions. On the other hand, physicians use certain techniques in an attempt to maintain their authority and control over the interaction: 1) the use of "overwhelming knowledge" to control the patient, 2) outlining negative consequences that may occur if the patient ignores their advice, and 3) personal appeal to the patient in a friendly manner. Koenig (2011) argues that when patients resist treatment recommendations, they are actively participating in the collaborative process, and thus forcing negotiations with physicians. In doing so, patients "assert their agency" and "collaboratively co-construct what counts as an acceptable recommendation" (p. 1105).

To this point, the discussion of the collaborative role of patients has focused on a single face-to-face interaction between a physician and a single patient. While this configuration is not uncommon, interactions can vary in both the number of visits and the number of participants. Significant others, such as family members and caretakers, may play an important role in collaboration when attending physicians' visits (Adelman, Greene and Charon, 1987). The presence of another nonexpert besides the patient creates an opportunity for coalitions to be formed. There may be multiple coalitions with different alignments during one interaction. These coalitions are fragile and fluid; a relative may enlist the help of the physician but not receive a response. Other times, a collocation may disband before the goal is reached (Coe and Prendergast 1985). The presence of a family member has also been shown to increase both the length of the visit and the amount of information that the physician shares with the patient (Labrecque et al., 1991). Much of the research on the collaborative effects of triads during physician visits focuses on elderly patients. Pediatric visits, however, are also fertile ground for studying the presence of a family member on interactions. Although there is a positive correlation between age of the child and his or her contribution to the interaction, children generally contribute relatively little to the collaborative process (Tates and Meeuwesen, 2001; Coyne, 2008).

Aside from multiple participants, physician–patient collaboration may include multiple interactions. Often, patients will maintain a continued dialog with their physicians that lasts multiple visits in an attempt to manage a disease that has already been diagnosed. This is especially true of individuals with chronic illnesses that may last a lifetime. In these cases, a new set of variables is introduced into the ongoing collaboration between patient and physician. As one example, some patients may choose to alter the prescribed treatment regimen. This is referred to as noncompliance within the medical profession. The label for this behavior is suggestive of the paternalistic mode of interaction that is still prevalent in the medical field. Instead of "adjusting," modifying," or even "correcting" medication timing or dosages, the patient is "noncompliant" and out of line with the instructions that were given by the physician. What physicians perceive as noncompliance, however, may be an attempt by the patient to exert control over his or her illness (Conrad, 1985). Whatever the label that is applied to this behavior, it is an example of the active role that patients take in determining the course of their treatment and more generally, entire illness experience. The alteration of treatment regimen is a unilateral act of agency when viewed in isolation. However, in the context of an ongoing, multi-visit physician consultation, the behavior demands response from the doctor (either acceptance or refutation) during the next visit. In this sense, the actions of patients outside of the physician's office are collaborative in that they alter the long-term strategy for disease management.

Collaborating on Diagnosis: Synthesizing Narratives

The aforementioned research on interactions and collaboration has been described in the context of treatment decisions. Decisions about treatment make up only a portion of the collaborative work between physicians and patients. Before treatment decisions are approached, a diagnosis must first be made. Despite the lack of attention to diagnosis in these models of interaction, the diagnostic process is extremely important. Brown (1995) efficiently summarizes the importance of diagnosis for both the patient and the physician:

> For patients, diagnosis can provide personal, emotional control, by way of knowing what is wrong. For medical professionals, diagnosis also provides control by mastering the knowledge of the problem at the individual care level. As well, diagnosis frequently determines the course of treatment ... For both patient and professional, diagnosis can lead to a prognosis. Physicians also employ diagnosis as a vehicle for building the whole body of medical knowledge.

Diagnosis marks the point at which all other subsequent interactions, decisions, and patient experiences are dependent. Without diagnosis, the physician cannot proceed with a course of treatment and the patient is not allowed to enter the sick role, thus legitimizing his illness experience. The sociology of diagnosis is a new subfield, and calls for more work in this area have already raised important questions regarding physician–patient collaboration during the diagnostic process (Brown, 1995; Jutel, 2009). Is there a space for collaboration during diagnosis, or is this phase of the clinical encounter simply a unilateral impartment of medical expertise upon the patient?

Early work on physician–patient interactions during the diagnostic process revealed little, if any, patient involvement (Heritage and Clayman, 2010). Diagnosis, which is not always delivered to the patient, is presented as an uncontestable fact and patients generally adopt a passive acceptance of the physician's ruling (Byrne, Long and Britain, 1976; Heath, 1992). Despite these findings, a growing body of research within medical sociology suggests that patients do, in fact, influence diagnosis during the interaction. Peräkylä (1998) presents a nuanced approach to understanding the balance between authority and accountability. The crux of this argument is that doctors do not rely on the authority granted to them that is prominent in the traditional "high physician agency" models discussed earlier. Instead, physicians "systematically make their diagnostic reasoning somewhat transparent for the patients, and thus treat themselves as accountable for the evidential basis of the diagnosis" (Peräkylä, 1998: 302). Peräkylä suggests that this new orientation toward accountability may be a function of the changing relationships between physicians and patients. The introduction of accountability into interactional models opens the door to patient agency within the diagnostic process. These findings and proposed explanation certainly parallel the newer models of physician–patient interactions that grant patients more autonomy and agency.

Interactions, both leading up to and during diagnosis, are often framed as discordant and some degree of tension may exist between the patient and physician regarding the expression of information and diagnostic hypotheses. Much of the disconnect between patients and physicians can be elucidated in the distinction between illness and disease (Eisenberg, 1977; Schneider and Conrad, 1981; Kleinman, Eisenberg and Good, 1978). Illness refers to the subjective, lived experience of the individual. Disease refers to the physiological state of dysfunction. This distinction between lived experience and physiological state is evident in the narratives that are expressed during the physician–patient interaction. The need for medical professionals to understand and account for these illness narratives as an expression of the lived experience of patients parallels the rise of chronic illness in modern societies (Bury, 2001; Kleinman, 1989). This rise in incidences of chronic illness requires physicians to account for the social, subjective experience of living with illness.

Despite the importance of integrating the patient narrative into the diagnostic process, it is the physician's narrative through which diagnosis is traditionally framed. This narrative is founded in, and an extension of, the biomedical gaze. The physician's narrative is one of objective rationalism. This objective, scientific approach is what lends legitimacy to a professional diagnosis, while at the same time, denying the subjective experiential narrative of the patient. The discord between these two narratives is the source of tension that is often a theme in research on the diagnostic process. Schneider and Conrad (1981) provide an illuminating example of these divergent narratives in their study of the different ways in which the experience of epilepsy is categorized by both patients and medical professionals. Medical typologies are delineated based on seizure pattern (e.g. grand mal versus petit mal). Patient typologies, however, reflect the social experience and impression management associated with living with and experiencing epilepsy in a social world. Patient typologies include categories such as "debilitated," "secret" and "pragmatic," which clearly signify different meanings than the medical typologies.

Ultimately, the diagnostic process is a marriage of both the patient's and physician's narratives. The degree to which the patient narrative is expressed and acknowledged is a determinant of the level of collaboration between physician and patient. In an ideally collaborative model, a rhetorical space must be carved out that allows for both narratives to find common ground. It is this "joint construction of narrative" (Brody, 1994) during the medical interviews that allows for the assignment of a diagnosis. As noted by Eggly (2002), "Narrative is not simply the telling of a chronological sequence of events by one speaker with the support ... of a listener; instead, the story is cocreated through the social interaction of the participants" (p. 350). These co-constructed narratives can take on multiple forms, including a discussion of the chronology of key events, repetition of key events, and most important to the discussion of diagnosis, the interpretation of key events (Eggly, 2002). It is this jointly constructed interpretation that should be a point of focus for future social science research on collaboration during diagnosis.

Gill and Maynard (2006) begin to address how these narratives are reconciled using conversational analysis. They reframe the tension between narratives (what they refer to as the "voice of medicine" and the "voice of the lifeworld") as "interactional dilemmas" that can be analyzed during clinical interactions between patients and physicians. Their argument is that this tension is a function of the "local, sequential organization of talk and the organization of the medical interview" (p. 147). They find that because of the structure of medical interviews, patients insert their own theories of diagnosis and etiology during the "data collection" phase. Patients use multiple techniques for introducing their explanations of illness into the conversation. While their research certainly suggests a tension that emerges from the structure of the interaction, it does not necessary preclude the presences of a larger tension between narratives. This type of analysis is just one of a myriad of approaches to understanding the collaborative techniques used by patients and physicians during the diagnostic process.

In the context of both diagnosis and treatment decisions, any complete analysis of health care collaboration should acknowledge the patient as possessing agency. Koenig (2011) provides a valuable discussion of patient agency during medical visits in his article on patient resistance in treatment decisions. He notes that "patient agency might be demonstrated by initiating an action, such as making a request for a particular kind of medical service" or "by responding to an action, such as the ways in which a patient's response to a treatment recommendation can begin a negotiation about the final treatment regime" (p. 1106). This distinction is important in that it acknowledges the subtle means by which patients navigate the power differential that exists in the physician–patient relationship. Agency can be enacted as a *response* to a physician request or suggestion. In recognizing that agency extends beyond explicit patient-initiated requests, the space for patient collaboration is greatly expanded. The importance of patient response as a reflection of agency is revealed in the work of Stivers (2005). Her work focuses on the reactions of parents in pediatric encounters and elucidates the ways in which parents can exert control over treatment through resistance. In order for treatment recommendation to come to a close, consensus must emerge. The initial response of the parents, be it explicit or covert, directs the course of the treatment decision-making process. Another example of enacting agency through reactions was mentioned earlier in this chapter. When patients alter their prescribed course of treatment (i.e. are noncompliant), they are also reacting to a physician's orders in a manner that affords them agency. Ultimately, whether it is during diagnostic judgments or treatment decisions, whether it is during face-to-face interactions or in the longer course of disease management, and whether it occurs through explicit suggestions or veiled resistance, patient agency has a constant presence in medical care.

Outcomes and Conclusion

Why does all of this matter? Just as with any collaborative work, be it benchside or bedside, the form that the collaborative interaction takes has an impact on the outcome of that collaborative effort. This is the impetus for many, if not most, studies on scientific collaboration—to understand how collaboration impacts performance, productivity, efficiency, etc. The same holds true for our understanding of physician–patient collaboration in clinical settings. The degree and type of collaboration during physician–patient interactions has been shown to impact health outcomes directly and indirectly. For example, Conboy et al. (2010) demonstrate that supportive physician–patient interactions lead to a decrease in self-reported IBS symptoms and an increased quality of life. This "supportive" interaction consisted of a holistic approach to patient collaboration, including a discussion of "emotional concerns, lifestyle questions, and exploration of the meaning of the disease for the subject" (p. 480). Note that these conversational elements strongly parallel the features of the patient narrative and perspective discussed in the previous section. Kaplan, Greenfield and Ware (1989) looked at specific facets of physician–patient communication and found that higher amounts of information provided by the physician, higher degree of patient control, and higher amounts of affect lead to better physiological health. A review of studies on physician–patient communication and health outcomes reveals that "effective" communication generally leads to improved outcomes (Stewart, 1995). Echoing the findings of the study above, Stewart (1995) states in her conclusion that,

> physicians should ask a wide range of questions, not only about physical aspects of the patients' problem, but also about his or her feelings and concerns, understanding of the problem, expectations about therapy, and perceptions of how the problem affects function. Patients need to feel that they are active participants in care ... (p. 1429)

Despite the support for the correlation between highly collaborative physician–patient interactions and positive physical health outcomes, the findings are not consistent throughout the literature. Some studies have found either no relationship or a negative relationship between the use of collaborative interactional techniques and physical health outcomes (Kinmonth et al., 1998; Bieber et al., 2006; Arora et al., 2009).

While findings on the effects of collaborative interactions on physical health are irregular, the effects of collaboration on other dimensions of patient care may be somewhat more consistent. Style of collaboration is associated with psychosocial and lifestyle variables such as patient satisfaction (Kinmonth et al., 1998), compliance and adherence (Kah et al., 2007; Arbuthnott and Sharpe, 2009), and coping (Bieber et al., 2006). These factors are important mediators in determining health outcomes. For example, when looking at the mental health of cancer survivors, Arora et al. (2009) found that physician styles that were more collaborative lead to increased patient self-efficacy and trust, which lead to increased sense of control and decreased uncertainty. These, in turn, lead to more positive mental health outcomes. Although some studies do find relationships between these dimensions of patient care, other studies that look at identical variables have nonsignificant results. In a review of the literature on patient-centered care and primary care outcomes, Mead and Bower (2002) concluded "the pattern of associations was not clear or consistent, and that some studies had shortcomings in terms of their internal and external validity" (p. 51). Most studies use patient satisfaction as the outcome variable of interest; these studies are "split in terms of relationships with satisfaction. Moreover, there are no obvious patterns in relation to other outcomes that have been studied" (p. 59). Harrington, Noble and Newman (2004) reviewed studies specifically on interventions that were intended to increase patient participation during medical consultations. Much like the Mead and Bower review (2002), results were inconsistent regarding outcome variables. For example, the meta-analysis showed that patient recall seems to be positively impacted by these interventions, but at the same time, there was no increase in the patients' knowledge of their illness (Harrington et al., 2004). Overall, we are left with an incomplete understanding of how patient participation and degree of collaboration impact health care outcomes, both physical and mental.

Of course, some of the inconsistences in the effects of type of collaboration on outcomes are due to the varying methodology and design of the studies (Mead and Bower, 2002).

But another way to explain the inconsistent findings in these studies mentioned above is that an important moderating variable has been generally ignored. A significant amount of research on the outcomes of collaboration and communication style do not account for patient preferences regarding type of collaboration. Concordance between patient preference and physician preference for medical collaboration is, in fact, a significant determinant of patient outcomes such as patient satisfaction and perceptions of health (Jahn et al., 2005). A meta-analysis of research on patient preferences found that overall, 63 percent of the studies showed that a majority (>50 percent) of respondents wanted to participate in decisions with their physician (Chewning et al., 2012). As one would expect, patient preferences regarding degree of collaboration and interaction style vary based on a number of variables. The health status of the study populations impacts patient preference outcomes. For example, in 77 percent of the studies that looked at cancer patients, the majority of patients preferred a more collaborative approach. However, in studies that looked at a general population of patients, only 53 percent of the studies showed a majority of patients wanting to participate, as opposed to letting the physician make decisions. Chewning et al. (2012) also found a temporal pattern in the research results; patient preference for participation in decision-making has increased over time. Demographic characteristics are also significant indicators of patient preferences. Swenson et al. (2004) report that, "Although most participants favored the patient-centered style, certain subgroups were less likely to prefer it … Older participants, participants with less formal education, and nonusers of CAM [complementary and alternative medicine] were significantly less likely than their counterparts to prefer the patient-centered doctor" (p. 1072). Given that patient preferences for collaboration matter in determining outcomes, and there is a high degree of variation in patient preferences, reaching an understanding of the relationship between preferences for collaboration, actual collaboration during the interaction, and outcomes, becomes challenging.

Research on understanding the moderating effects of patient preferences on the relationship between degree of collaboration and outcomes is sparse, but not completely lacking. Lee and Lin (2010) performed a longitudinal study of Taiwanese diabetes patients that examined the potential for the moderating effects of patient preferences for autonomy on the relationship between physician support for autonomy and outcomes. There was some support for this moderating effect, but the results raise more questions. For example, patient preference regarding the receipt of comprehensive information was a significant moderator of self-assessed physical and mental health outcomes, but its moderating effects were nonsignificant in predicting physiological indicators of increased health. At the same time, patient preference for involvement in decision-making was nonsignificant as a moderating effect on both self-assessed health and physiological markers of health. The Yang and Lin (2010) study paints a complex picture of the relationship between patient preferences for collaboration with the physician, degree of collaboration during an interaction, and health outcomes. The multidimensional aspects of collaboration (both preferred and enacted) and outcomes (physical and mental) make this area of research particularly difficult. As such, there is still much to be done to inform our understanding of the relationships between these variables.

Physician patient collaboration is integral to our understanding of collaboration in the health sciences. While it is clear that form of interaction and degree of collaboration that occurs between physicians and patients varies significantly, the outcomes of these different collaborative forms has yet to be understood. Patients enter the physician visit with preconceived ideas regarding their illness experience and possible diagnostic and treatment options. The presentation of symptoms and illness history, the act of diagnosis, and discussion of treatment options are all potentially collaborative moments involving the active patient. During face-to-face interactions, patients collaborate by presenting their own lived experience to the physician and negotiating diagnosis and treatment. Decisions are reached based on a fusion of personal understanding and expert knowledge. The recognition of illness narratives as still existing outside of the scientific cannon, but nonetheless, being a necessary component of competent doctoring denotes a willingness to collaborate with patients. Physicians and medical professionals may still draw clear lines of demarcation between expert and lay knowledge as a means to maintain professional authority and sovereignty, but they do build bridges between their world of professional knowledge and the world of lived experiences of lay individuals. These bridges, some of which I hope to have exposed in this chapter, are the points of partnership that deserve attention in research on collaboration.

The purpose of this chapter was to introduce patients as active agents in collaborative processes in the practice of medicine. Theories and research on different forms of physician–patient interaction and collaboration have been synthesized and summarized in the hopes that these theories provide readers, who may not otherwise be exposed to this body of literature, an opportunity to think about lay individuals as collaborative agents. Much of the STS research focuses on collaboration between professionals and a smaller portion of the literature examines collaboration be professionals and nonprofessionals at the institutional and organizational level. However, the individual patient must also be acknowledged as a collaborative agent in the health care process.

References

Adelman, R.D., Greene, M.G. and Charon, R. 1987. The physician-elderly patient-companion triad in the medical encounter: The development of a conceptual framework and research agenda. *The Gerontologist*, 27(6), 729–34.

Arbuthnott, A. and Sharpe, D. 2009. The effect of physician–patient collaboration on patient adherence in non-psychiatric medicine. *Patient Education and Counseling*, 77(1), 60–67.

Arora, N.K., Weaver, K.E., Clayman, M.L., Oakley-Girvan, I. and Potosky, A.L. 2009. Physicians' decision-making style and psychosocial outcomes among cancer survivors. *Patient Education and Counseling*, 77(3), 404–12.

Bieber, C., Muller, K.G., Blumenstiel, K., et al. 2006. Long-term effects of a shared decision-making intervention on physician–patient interaction and outcome in fibromyalgia. A qualitative and quantitative 1 year follow-up of a randomized controlled trial. *Patient Education and Counseling*, 63(3), 357–66.

Bissell, P., May, C.R. and Noyce, P.R. 2004. From compliance to concordance: Barriers to accomplishing a re-framed model of health care interactions. *Social Science and Medicine*, 58(4), 851–62.

Brody, H. 1994. My story is broken; can you help me fix it? Medical ethics and the joint construction of narrative. *Literature and Medicine*, 13(1), 79–92.

Brown, P. 1995. Naming and framing: The social construction of diagnosis and illness. *Journal of Health and Social Behavior*, 25, 34–52.

Bucchi, M. and Neresini, F. 2008. Science and public participation. *The Handbook of Science and Technology Studies*. Cambridge, MA: MIT Press, 449–72.

Bury, M. 2001. Illness narratives: Fact or fiction? *Sociology of Health and Illness*, 23(3), 263–85.

Byrne, P.S., Long, B.E.L. and Britain, G. 1976. *Doctors Talking to Patients: A Study of the Verbal Behaviour of General Practitioners Consulting in Their Surgeries*, HM Stationery Office.

Charles, C., Gafni, A. and Whelan, T. 1999. Decision-making in the physician–patient encounter: Revisiting the shared treatment decision-making model. *Social Science and Medicine*, 651–61.

Charles, C., Gafni, A. and Whelan, T. 1997. Shared decision-making in the medical encounter: What does it mean? (Or it takes at least two to tango). *Social Science and Medicine*, 44, 681–92.

Chewning, B., Bylund, C.L., Shah, B., Arora, N.K., Gueguen, J.A. and Makoul, G. 2012. Patient preferences for shared decisions: A systematic review. *Patient Education and Counseling*, 86(1), 9–18.

Chin, J.J. 2002. Doctor–patient relationship: From medical paternalism to enhanced autonomy. *Singapore Medical Journal*, 43(3), 152–5.

Coe, R.M. and Prendergast, C.G. 1985. The formation of coalitions: Interaction strategies in triads. *Sociology of Health and Illness*, 7(2), 236–47.

Conboy, L., Macklin, E.A., Kelly, J., et al. 2010. Which patients improve: Characteristics increasing sensitivity to a supportive patient–practitioner relationship. *Social Science and Medicine*, 70(3), 479–84.

Conrad, P. 1985. The meaning of medications: Another look at compliance. *Social Science and Medicine*, 20(1), 29–37.

Coyne, I. 2008. Children's participation in consultations and decision-making at health service level: A review of the literature. *International Journal of Nursing Studies*, 45(11), 1682.

Eggly, S. 2002. Physician–patient co-construction of illness narratives in the medical interview. *Health Communication*, 14(3), 339–60.

Eisenberg, L. 1977. Disease and illness. Distinctions between professional and popular ideas of sickness. *Culture, Medicine and Psychiatry*, 1(1), 9–23.

Emanuel, E.J. and Emanuel, L.L. 2000. Four models of the physician–patient relationship. *Readings in Health Care Ethics*, 1, 40–49.

Epstein, S. 2008. Patient groups and health movements. *The Handbook of Science and Technology Studies*. Cambridge, MA: MIT Press, 449.

Eysenbach, G. and Jadad, A.R. 2001. Evidence-based patient choice and consumer health informatics in the Internet age. *Journal of Medical Internet Research*, 3(2), e19.

Ford, S., Schofield, T. and Hope, T. 2003. What are the ingredients for a successful evidence-based patient choice consultation? A qualitative study. *Social Science and Medicine*, 56(3), 589.

Gill, V.T. and Maynard, D.W. 2006. Explaining illness: Patients' proposals and physicians' responses. *Studies in Interactional Sociolinguistics*, 20, 115.

Hackett, E.J. 2005. Introduction to the special guest-edited issue on 'Scientific Collaboration'. *Social Studies of Science*, 35, 667–71.

Haug, M.R. and Lavin, B. 1981. Practitioner or patient—who's in charge? *Journal of Health and Social Behavior*, 22(3), 212–29.

Hayes-Bautista, D.E. 1976. Modifying the treatment: Patient compliance, patient control and medical care. *Social Science and Medicine*, 10(5), 233–8.

Heath, C. 1992. The delivery and reception of diagnosis in the general-practice consultation, *Talk at Work: Interaction in Institutional Settings*, 8, 235–67.

Heritage, J. and Clayman, S. 2010. *Talk in Action: Interactions, Identities, and Institutions*. Wiley-Blackwell.

Hope, T. 1999. Evidence-based patient choice. *Evidence Based Medicine*, 4(2), 38–40.

Jahng, K.H., Martin, L.R., Golin, C.E. and DiMatteo, M.R. 2005. Preferences for medical collaboration: Patient–physician congruence and patient outcomes. *Patient Education and Counseling*, 57(3), 308.

Jutel, A. 2009. Sociology of diagnosis: A preliminary review. *Sociology of Health and Illness*, 31(2), 278–99.

Kahn, K.L., Schneider, E., Malin, J.L., Adams, J.L. and Epstein, A.M. 2007. Patient centered experiences in breast cancer: Predicating long-term adherence to tamoxifen use. *Medical Care*, 45(5), 431–9.

Kaplan, S.H., Greenfield, S. and Ware, J.E.Jr. 1989. Assessing the effects of physician–patient interactions on the outcomes of chronic disease. *Medical Care*, 27(3), S110–27.

Kasteler, J., Kane, R.L., Olsen, D.M. and Thetford, C. 1976. Issues underlying prevalence of doctor-shopping behavior. *Journal of Health and Social Behavior,* 17(4), 328–39.

Kinmonth, A.L, Woodcock, A., Griffin, S., Spiegal, N. and Campbell, M.J. 1998. Randomised controlled trial of patient centred care of diabetes in general practice: Impact on current wellbeing and future disease risk. *British Medical Journal*, 317(7167), 1202–8.

Kleinman, A. 1989. *The Illness Narratives: Suffering, Healing, and the Human Condition*, Basic Books.

Kleinman, A., Eisenberg, L. and Good, B. 1978. Culture, illness, and care: Clinical lessons from anthropologic and cross-cultural research. *Annals of Internal Medicine*, 88(2), 251.

Koenig, C.J. 2011. Patient resistance as agency in treatment decisions. *Social Science and Medicine*, 72(7), 1105–14.

Labrecque, M.S., Blanchard, C.G., Ruckdeschel, J.C. and Blanchard, E.B. 1991. The impact of family presence on the physician–cancer patient interaction. *Social Science and Medicine*, 33(11), 1253–61.

Lee, Y. and Lin, J.L. 2010. Do patient autonomy preferences matter? Linking patient-centered care to patient–physician relationships and health outcomes. *Social Science and Medicine*, 71, 1811–18.

Levine, M.N., Gafni, A., Markham, B. and MacFarlane, D. 1992. A bedside decision instrument to elicit a patient's preference concerning adjuvant chemotherapy for breast cancer. *Annals of Internal Medicine*, 117(1), 53.

Makoul, G. and Clayman, M.L. 2006. An integrative model of shared decision making in medical encounters. *Patient Education and Counseling*, 60(3), 301.

Marinker, M. and Sharp, M. 1997. *From Compliance to Concordance: Achieving Shared Goals in Medicine Taking.* Royal Pharmaceutical Society of Great Britain and Merck Sharp and Dohme.

McKinlay, J.B. and Marceau, L.D. 2002. The end of the golden age of doctoring. *International Journal of Health Services*, 32(2), 379–416.

Mead, N. and Bower, P. 2002. Patient-centered consultations and outcomes in primary care: A review of the literature. *Patient Education and Counseling*, 48, 51–61.

Moumjid, N., Gafni, A., Bremond, A. and Carrere, M.O. 2007. Shared decision making in the medical encounter: Are we all talking about the same thing? *Medical Decision Making*, 27(5), 539–46.

Parsons, T. 1951. *The Social System.* Psychology Press.

Perakyla, A. 1998. Authority and accountability: The delivery of diagnosis in primary health care. *Social Psychology Quarterly*, 61(4), 301–20.

Quill, T.E. and Brody, H. 1996. Physician recommendations and patient autonomy: Finding a balance between physician power and patient choice. *Annals of Internal Medicine*, 125(9), 763.

Reeder, L.G. 1972. The patient-client as a consumer: Some observations on the changing professional–client relationship. *Journal of Health and Social Behavior*, 13(4), 406–12.

Safran, D.G., Montgomery, J.E., Chang, H., Murphy, J. and Rogers, W.H. 2001. Switching doctors: Predictors of voluntary disenrollment from a primary physician's practice. *Journal of Family Practice*, 50(2), 130–36.

Schneider, J.W. and Conrad, P. 1981. Medical and sociological typologies: The case of epilepsy. *Social Science and Medicine*, 15(3), 211–19.

Sebban, C., Browman, G., Gafni, A., Norman, G., Levine, M., Assouline, D. and Fiere, D. 1995. Design and validation of a bedside decision instrument to elicit a patient's preference concerning allogenic bone marrow transplantation in chronic myeloid leukemia. *American Journal of Hematology*, 48(4), 221–7.

Starr, P. 1984. *The Social Transformation of American Medicine: The Rise of a Sovereign Profession and the Making of a Vast Industry.* Basic Books.

Stewart, M.A. 1995. Effective physician–patient communication and health outcomes: A review. *Canadian Medical Association Journal*, 152(9), 1423–33.

Stivers, T. 2005. Parent resistance to physicians' treatment recommendations: One resource for initiating a negotiation of the treatment decision. *Health Communication*, 18(1), 41–74.

Sullivan, T. (ed.) 1998. *Collaboration: A Health Care Imperative.* McGraw-Hill.

Swenson, S.L., Buell, S., Zettler, P., White, M., Ruston, D.C. and Lo, B. 2004. Patient-centered communication: Do patients really prefer it? *Journal of General Internal Medicine*, 19(11), 1069.

Szasz, T.S. and Hollender, M.H. 1956. A contribution to the philosophy of medicine: The basic models of the doctor-patient relationship. *Archives of Internal Medicine*, 97(5), 585.

Tates, K. and Meeuwesen, L. 2001. Doctor–parent–child communication. A (re)view of the literature. *Social Science and Medicine*, 52(6), 839–51.

Veatch, R.M. 1972. Models for ethical medicine in a revolutionary age. *Hastings Center Report*, 5–7.

Weissman, J.S., Blumenthal, D., Silk, A.J., Newman, M., Zapert, K., Leitman, R. and Feibelmann, S. 2004. Physicians report on patient encounters involving direct-to-consumer advertising. *Health Affairs*, 23, 292.

PART V
Conclusion

Chapter 11

The Health of Collaborations: A Reflection

Andrew Webster

Introduction

The UK Higher Education system conducts an evaluation exercise every five years to determine the quality of research activity in universities, on the basis of which the subsequent allocation of government research funding is determined. Similar models and approaches are found elsewhere, indeed some copying the UK model. However, the most recent exercise, in 2013/14, yet to report its results, introduced a new metric through which quality is to be judged: alongside publications, numbers of PhDs and grant income won, those submitting had to include 'impact case studies' showing how their research had some sort of tractable outcome or impact on its end users. In February 2014, the first high-level data emerging from the exercise, the Research Excellence Framework (REF), reported that 6,975 impact cases had been included in the overall submission to the UK government agency handling the review, a submission which comprised 52,077 staff and 191,232 research outputs (HEFCE, 2014).

Many of these case studies will be built on collaboration narratives involving diverse forms of engagement between researchers and research users, public and private actors, and the third sector, with many anchored in health research. An audit trail had to be provided with the case studies to show how research users were involved in, directly collaborated with, and so derived some tangible benefit from the research. Proving impact requires proving collaboration, and increasingly, the turn towards 'co-production' (Pohl, 2008). Most commentaries on the REF have framed it very much in terms of audit and evaluation and the growing metricisation of the academy (e.g. Kelly and Burrows, 2012), pointing to both the pathologies of and gaming associated with this. But, notwithstanding this, it is also important to note the way the mantra of impact drives research to being 'strategic', collaborative and increasingly applied, not simply between disciplines but also between academic and non-academic sectors. This in turn leads to the move towards larger interdisciplinary research projects and networks, and growing complexity over the nature of 'the problem' to be addressed, and what thereby might count as a 'solution'. This has become even more demanding as a result of the rapid development of, access to and drive towards mining large data sets – so-called 'big data'. Added layers of complexity appear as the data is then processed through, for example, integrated agent-based multi-scale simulations, coupled with large-scale data streaming engines.

For those constructing their impact cases for the REF, the problem is always finding a narrative about collaboration which is linear, directly causal and well-planned, though some serendipity is allowed to figure too. It is on this basis that best practice guides to and 'road-maps' for collaboration are produced and disseminated. As the chapters of this book show however, collaborative activity between disciplines and sectors, even that which is carefully planned and resourced, has not only different and often competing interests at work, but is highly non-linear, iterative and uncertain in its effects and value. None of these chapters could have been the basis for a tidy impact case study. Much would have to have been left out or a veil drawn over the more difficult parts. For example, Schleifer's chapter which explores collaboration between Unilever and Dutch food scientists about 'trans fats', shows, paradoxically, that it was only by doubting the scientists claims about these fats that the industry moved towards replacing trans fats in margarine. Here, impact results from dismissal. These chapters all throw light on the performativity of collaboration and co-production and crucially, how this shapes what counts as producing knowledge which is seen to have value – or perhaps not so when it concerns a trans fat. In this brief commentary I want to offer some reflections on what the book tells us about forms of collaboration and the implications this has for wider debates especially about health research, evidence and transitions in the science system.

The Implications of New Forms of Collaboration

Collaborative research is, in itself, nothing new. In their very different ways, Merton (1973), Hagstrom (1965) and subsequently, those writing much later from an actor network theory (ANT) perspective (Latour, 1987; Law and Hassard, 1999) highlight the ways in which the construction, validation and mobilisation of knowledge depends on others – on 'the scientific community' in the first case, and on heterogeneous actors and 'actants' in the second. The chapters in this book, however, speak to a qualitative shift in the ways in which epistemic communities and their networks are configured, in general, and specifically in the field of health-related research and practice, building on earlier work in the sciences (Parker et al., 2010). The contributions by Merton and others were primarily or at least often have been (in the case of ANT) focused on collaboration within discrete scientific domains, within a specific scientific landscape. The chapters here chart a very diverse, complex and often highly unstable meaning as to who is a collaborator and who is not, with their diversity characterised in almost churchly terms as 'large congregations' (see Helgesson and Krafve) from all quarters of the health universe. What do we learn about these new forms of collaboration?

First, a number of the chapters identify the ever-expanding scale – professional, disciplinary, organisational and geographical – of collaboration seen today, characterised by a complex division of intellectual labour. Mattsson, for example, in a detailed exploration of bibliometric data describes how health research is becoming increasingly interdisciplinary and trans-institutional in the 'bench-to-bedside' process, as producers and users try to put into practice 'translational medicine'. Different sources and forms of expertise are seen to be needed not simply to undertake research but to apply it, and this can be best orchestrated through large scale projects. Mattsson's patterns of co-authorship will often map onto large-scale projects, and it is the latter which Vermeulen's concept of 'projectification' seeks to emphasise in her study of the VIRGO network. The advent of the now ubiquitous 'Workpackage' and its associated 'deliverables' in research projects ensures that research can be managed across diverse groups and interests – here industrial and academic – while each retains a specific, discrete responsibility and intellectual home in which they feel comfortable. It is perhaps then not surprising that next to the scientific 'quality' of a bid, considerable weight is given to its management, or the co-ordination of the actor network where discrete interests can be mobilised and where possible integrated. How deliverables are framed is crucial to shaping the nature of the collaboration and the clauses of the formal agreement that polices all project members. Do some deliverables – such as patents – as in the VIRGO case, drive the project overall and determine the nature of collaboration, or is there space for others, and can ingenuity, serendipity and the exploration of 'areas of ignorance' (Mulkay, 1990) even be a 'deliverable'? This highlights one of the trade-offs of collaboration where on the one hand we see the tendency of large networks towards closure and standardisation while on the other once can ask how does this meet the need to retain space for innovation at a local level?

Standardisation is driven by and configures the scale and utility of integrative technology platforms that characterise large-scale science. The Human Genome Project was perhaps the most iconic example of this but today bioinformatics systems are commonplace across molecular, epigenomic and stem cell research fields. Standards not only set the ontological boundaries – or divisions – of the biomedical tissues found in these fields but act to police, audit and certify contributions and contributors to the field itself. Standardisation is then primarily an epistemic and a filtering endeavour (Busch, 2011). The chapter by Helgesson and Krafve provides a very nuanced commentary on a particular form of standardising found in health collaborations, the clinical registry. Whereas most standardising processes seek by definition to reduce heterogeneity and contingency, clinical registries pose problems here as they are large data sets generated by a wide variety of biomedical researchers and clinicians that carry a diverse range of information. The authors show how the registries might be drawn on to secure patients for clinical trials in the area of rare disease, a field of inquiry where trials of patient populations are notoriously difficult to mount given the problems of defining the boundaries and specific conditions of rare diseases and so which patients should be included and excluded. Ironically, however, since the conventional, 'gold standard' clinical trial model (Will and Moreria, 2010) requires a double-blind design the actual contribution a trial makes to understanding a rare disease might be limited: as Helgesson and Krafve argue, '… [it is] difficult to enter data about the treatment in the registry form, precisely since this information is blinded during the course of the trial' (p. 117).

Secondly, the chapters not only describe the scale and the relationship between the structuring of research and the epistemic spaces opened up or closed down by collaboration, they also point to the ways in which funding is driving collaboration. The principal driver behinds this appears in a number of the chapters: this is how the structuring of research funding not merely incentivises but requires collaboration (as we see in the European Commission's Horizon 2020 programme, for example, where proposals must include both public and private sector actors) and indeed is rewarded for it: a lone scholar is often very much alone. This development, seen over the last decade in particular, raises questions over the ways in which top-down, interventionist funding programmes rewrite the norms on which academic research is to be conducted and regulated (Benner and Sandstrom, 2000). Increasingly, these norms are geared more to serving commercial interests: as Vermeulen observes, in the VIRGO projects the focus shifted from academic publications to results that fit into the industrial mode of ordering aiming for patents (p. 54).

Thirdly, it is especially interesting to reflect on this matter of normative regulation a little more since as the chapters show, given the scale of collaboration – in terms of funding, co-authorship, transnational networks and so on, we can ask where the locus of responsibility lies in regard to managing error, accountability for evidence, sign-off of results and the processes and structures through which reward is given to different biomedical science groups. Intellectual property rights can be especially difficult to manage and allocate across large scale projects (Hilgartner, 2012) not least in determining claims over background rights that preceded the collaboration compared with foreground rights that emerged as a result of new knowledge or techniques created as a result of the collaboration. This in turn raises questions about the ownership of an access to data. More generally, returning to the world of Mertonian norms and its rewards and sanctions, what do norms and sanctions mean here in managing deviance and rewarding success in science in such large networks? How are deviance and success defined, identified, and policed, especially in health research involving diverse and often competing interests, and the ever-present pressure 'to deliver'. And how do these in turn relate to the ways in which scientists use their social capital, as discussed by Mikami earlier in this book in his discussion of regenerative medicine in Japan. There are then different types of reward (and sanction) cultures operating in science reflecting the use and recognition of different claims to authority and to value of work done – in terms of novelty, utility, intellectual property and more broadly based professional capital – that may coalesce, be diluted, or work in different directions in the world of large-scale collaboration.

At the same time, it is important to be wary of overstating the centrifugal tendencies of large networks in health or other fields since there are always competing tendencies towards the local inasmuch as local expertise, technical resources, datasets and the specific scientific capital a centre or research group enjoys in a field are the very basis on which engagement in collaboration is offered and secured. In addition, the scientific value of a collaborative network is not only realised at a consortium level but also in more localised settings. In their analysis of large-scale sequencing, Davies et al. (2013) show that labs are keen to participate precisely because they hope to be able to 'integrate and reuse the data available online for their own research purposes'. This localisation is also reinforced in health research as Mattsson shows in her chapter on trials. She argues that while trans-institutional collaboration is common this is more likely to be geographically local to a specific region because of the contingencies of health care systems, and their particular procurement, ethical cultures, and reimbursement regimes. Finally, Lewin's discussion of the active role of patients in developing a collaborative diagnosis and treatment with physicians stresses the importance of localised and indeed individualised patient cultures that provide an understanding of illness experiences and which inform patient outcomes precisely because of the sort of collaboration with clinicians that they experience.

Platforms Enabling Collaboration

A significant characteristic of the science system today is the growth of large-scale 'platforms' that support and align national and international networks, and might be seen as the defining feature of contemporary 'research infrastructures' (Shinn and Marcovich, 2012). These platforms are associated with the growth of digital technologies, especially bioinformatics which allows the creation of databases – 'Big Data' – and the means to interrogate them. The scale at which biomedical data manipulation can be undertaken to support new health research is such that conventional data/disciplinary boundaries are disturbed as the level of data aggregation allows new possibilities (such as in regard to the storage and preservation of information or tissue in biobanks for example) and so new interpretation of the data to be made.

How do these new biomedical data sets and their results relate to the equally large public health data, personal e-health records and service-related administrative data sets that government agencies and institutions are responsible for? Typically, very poorly, which is why there has been a recent push to mobilise the latter in order to add value to the former: in the UK, for example, the government Department of Health via NHS England has recently proposed to gather patient records to create a new data repository holding patients' medical histories, information which would then be available to third parties undertaking biomedical research (in both the public and private sectors) as well as insurance companies. This was one form of 'healthy collaboration' which turned out to be politically unhealthy because of concerns over consent and access by third parties to private information. The proposal was put on ice, sharing thereby a political version of the fate met by tissue samples in biobanks (Kirby, 2014)

Moreover, notwithstanding such developments, agencies and institutions responsible for health services (or other socio-technical sectors such as transport, utilities and education) are increasingly fragmented in terms of data sharing and governance structures. This is a common feature of healthcare systems in Europe that have witnessed the privatisation of public services, public cut backs, and a changing and changeable architecture of policy making, in part driven by the neo-liberal turn. Different agencies collect different sorts of data and intelligence about health, but often do not share that intelligence across the sector or actors. This also means that the relationship between health science and policy has become increasingly *politicised* and *socially distributed* (across quangos, advisory agencies, NGOs, learned bodies, regulatory bodies, etc.). Hence, the relationship between evidence and the three principal areas of health policy making – strategy, policy development and policy delivery – is complex, and non-linear (Bielak et al., 2008). At the same time, policy implementation depends on an understanding of the receptivity of those whom it is supposed to affect. The merits of a particular health policy intervention based on the results of biomedical research are often measured by cost-benefit assessments in terms of tangible outcomes, precisely because it is assumed that these do not depend on interpretive judgement. However, as the discussion by Lecluijze et al. in Chapter 7 shows, it is often the case that interpretations of evidence – evidence which they describe as 'scripts' – can vary considerably across social actors as can the merits of particular outcome measures (Armstrong, 2009). It is equally, perhaps more, important therefore to understand the *social* platforms that make technology platforms workable.

The spread of open source platforms, crowd sourcing, real-time data scraping, web-based data collection (webdatametrics) and, in terms of the evaluation of scientific research, 'altmetrics' (that use social media activity – such as blogs etc. – as an alternative set of markers of reputation to the conventional peer review assessment of scientists' work) are generating radically different processes and criteria through which evidentiaries are being built and given value. These developments also change the social geography of collaboration (Hinchlifffe, 2007) opening up new loci within which very different voices are heard and which require very different coordinative action to make them heard within the conventional circles and halls of established science. The spatial practices of health science are given only limited attention in the chapters except for that by Vermeulen who speaks of the 'spatial orderings' of the VIRGO network and the redrawing of boundaries within it. Understanding the articulation between technological, social and open platforms will be the key to future work in social science on the collaborative dynamics of knowledge not simply in the field of health but elsewhere too.

Collaboration between the Health and Social Sciences

A final theme which the chapters by Albert et al. and Mesman explore is the ways in which social science is positioned as co-producer in collaborative research programmes, the authors recounting their quite different experiences of this. The chapter by Albert et al. provides a very useful account of the range of views held by bioscientists and clinicians in regard to the value of social science, principally of qualitative research. The boundary work done by scientists and to a slightly lesser extent by clinicians produces a hierarchy of knowledge that privileges the experimental approach and discounts qualitative work as 'research' as such; even quantitative social science is seen in a hand-maiden role, since such work does not in itself have a direct interventional set of outcomes on health care because it can only deal in correlations not causes. These arguments are of course spoken from a position of relative ignorance of the actual contribution that, say, public health social science has made to bring about – to cause – improvements in general health of a population (Graham, 2012). The authors argue that more exposure to social science helps to overcome such resistances. What is likely to make this exposure more productive here is the ways in which social science can create a shared methodological problem with the sciences – say over how best to understand the process through which patient interpretation of clinical conditions shapes their response to medical treatment and the impact this has on the management of these specific conditions. Patient concordance, for example, to a drugs regime which is directly supported by biomedical evidence, might well depend in practice on patients' localised understanding of the efficacy and value of medicines: much of the time these will overlap with the views of physicians but where and why they do not is a crucial issue that crosses the biomedical/social science divide and demands attention from both (Webster et al., 2009).

Equally importantly, Mesman's chapter that discusses over 20 years' experience observing *neonatal intensive care units* shows how a social science understanding of the performativity of clinical science and practice along with what she calls engagement with an '*organizational form of work*', produces a collaborative dynamic which is highly productive and which as a result dissolves the discrete lines, the trading zones, between the researched and the researcher, between the clinicians and the social scientist, leading to what she calls a specific form of understanding, 'collaborative knowledge'. The use of visual technologies as a medium for reflecting on practice repositioned all parties as part of the same scene and so as co-actors in the hospital and acted as a vehicle for co-production of knowledge and a change in practice.

There are lessons from both these chapters about effective social science collaboration. What is evident is that trans-disciplinarity is difficult to achieve when sought through epistemic alignment but easier to achieve when, ironically, it is not explicitly pursued. Instead exposure and immersion (as in Mesman's case) appears to create a different sort of space for engagement. There have been recent debates in science and technology studies about the form and degree of engagement with the practitioners of science (Webster, 2007) and how to retain a critical perspective, especially in regard to science policy. It seems likely that the lessons from this book about health(y) collaboration could and should be drawn on by social science. So as social scientists it would be possible to play a key role in understanding the ways in which a socio-technical platform might be built to enable more effective health research and delivery; to show how such platforms have to rethink the roles of knowledge, situated practices and measures for evaluating outcomes; and finally, while knowledge networks are key to responding to contemporary societal challenges these networks are not established in some 'natural' way but have multiple possible intellectual trajectories and cross diverse institutional boundaries. Securing links with decision-makers in local or wider settings is likely to be key to the take-up of results as will the provision of what are seen as robust models and associated socio-technical interventions, such as the normalisation process 'tool-kit' developed by May and others (May, 2009) which has been adopted widely in healthcare.

Conclusion

These brief reflections on the themes that are encompassed by the various chapters of this book suggest that there are some important developments in health research and practice in terms of scale, geography, locus of authority and measures of what counts as good evidence and good practice. The shifts might be seen as part of a wider transition in the science system within and beyond health itself. A recent rather programmatic statement has been published by a group of Dutch STS scholars (Dijstelbloem et al., 2013) that argues that the world of science is characterised by rapid rates of publication, globalised networks of research, increasingly expensive equipment and, as a result, the need to produce more data whose quality is open to question, and where the ability to check for data massaging or indeed fraud itself is made more difficult. Ironically, the scale of these networks is said to work against effective communication of scientific results. The chapters here point to the dangers of collaboration as well as the new possibilities that are opened up by it. The dark-side of collaboration – its more unhealthy form – is at least as important to recognise and discuss as is its more healthy variant.

Finally, to return to another classic, Kuhn (1977) this time, is it the case that today's 'normal science' is 'collaborative science'? If so, and if marked by what has been sketched out above and elsewhere in the book, what would or could constitute 'revolutionary' science? Are there no longer paradigmatic forms of knowledge that can be disrupted by 'breakthrough' since trans-disciplinarity and global science networks are forever geared towards iterative rather than radical shifts in understanding that move on different fronts at the same time. This might create problems for creativity (Nowotny, 2008) and will make the 'application' of knowledge more complex. It will require new trans-institutional structures that will be able to realise the benefits of this form of knowledge, but ones which we currently do not have.

References

Armstrong, D. 2009. Stabilising the construct of health-related quality of life: 1970–2007. *Science Studies*, 22(2), 102–15.

Benner, M. and Sandstrom, L. 2000. Institutionalizing the triple helix: Research funding and norms in the academic system. *Research Policy*, 29(1), 291–301.

Bielak, A., Campbell, A., Pope, S., Schaefer K. and Shaxson, L. 2008. From science communications to knowledge brokering: The shift from 'science push' to 'policy pull'. In: Cheng, D., Claessens, M., Gascoigne, T., Metcalfe, J. and Schiele, B. (eds) *Communicating Science in Social Contexts: New Models, New Practices*. New York: Springer, 201–26.

Busch, L. 2011. *Standards. Recipes for Reality*. Boston: MIT Press.

Dijstelbloem, H., Huisman, F., Miedema, F., Ravetz, J. and Mijnhardt, W. 2013. Science in transition: Utrecht. Report, http://www.scienceintransition.nl/english.

Graham, H. 2014. Cutting down: Insights from qualitative studies of smoking in pregnancy. *Health and Social Care in the Community*, 22, 259–67.

Hagstrom, W.O. 1965. *The Scientific Community*. New York: Basic Books.

HEFCE 2014. Review of REF Submissions. Higher Education Funding Council for England. London: HMSO.

Hilgartner, S. 2012. Selective flows of knowledge in technoscientific interaction: Information control in genome research. *The British Journal for History of Science*, 45, 1–14.

Hinchliffffe, S. 2007. *Geographies of Nature*. Milton Keynes: Open University Press.

Kelly, A. and Burrows, R. 2012. Measuring the value of sociology? Some notes on the performative metricisation of the contemporary academy. In: L. Adkins & C. Lury (eds) *Measure and Value: A Sociological Review Monograph*. Oxford: Wily-Blackwell, 130–50.

Kirby, T. 2014. Controversy surrounds England's new NHS database. *The Lancet*, 383(9918), 681.

Kuhn, T. 1977. *The Essential Tension: Selected Studies in Scientific Tradition and Change*. Chicago and London: University of Chicago Press.

Latour, B. 1987. *Science in Action: How to Follow Scientists and Engineers Through Society*. Milton Keynes: Open University Press.

Law, J. and Hassard, J. (eds) 1999. *Actor Network Theory and After*. Oxford and Keele: Blackwell and the Sociological Review.

May, C. 2009. Innovation and implementation in health technology: Normalizing telemedicine. In: J. Gabe and M. Calnan (eds) *The New Sociology of the Health Service*. London: Routledge, 143–60.

Merton, R. 1973. *The Sociology of Science*. Chicago: Chicago University Press.

Mulkay, M. 1990. *Sociology of Science: A Sociological Pilgrimage*. Milton Keynes: Open University Press.

Nowotny, H. 2008. *Insatiable Curiosity: Innovation in a Fragile Future*. Cambridge Massachusetts: The MIT Press.

Parker, J.N., Vermeulen, N. and Penders, B. (eds) 2010. *Collaboration in the New Life Sciences*. Aldershot: Ashgate.

Pohl, C. 2008. From science to policy through transdisciplinary research. *Environmental Science and Policy*, 11, 46–53.

Shinn, T. and Marcovich, A. 2012. Regimes of science production and diffusion: Towards a transverse organization of knowledge. *Scientiae Studia*, 10, 33–64.

Webster, A. 2007. Crossing boundaries: STS in the policy room. *Science, Technology and Human Values*, 32, 458–78.

Webster, A., Douglas, C. and Lewis, G. 2009. Making sense of medicines. *Science as Culture*, 18, 233–47.

Will, C. and Moreira, T. (eds) 2010. *Medical Proofs and Social Experiments*. Durham: Durham University Press.

Index